Finding Solid Footing: Thriving Beyond the Unimaginable

By Katy Grainger

Cover design by Andrea Schmidt

Cover Photos by Nani Welch Keli`iho`omalu

Hair and Makeup by Tia Yagi

ISBN - Amazon Hardcover: 979-8-9953590-0-5

ISBN - Paperback: 979-8-9953590-1-2

PRAISE FOR FINDING SOLID FOOTING

"In her powerful and inspiring new book, Katy Grainger brings to life, in vivid, heart-wrenching detail, her experience as a sepsis victim, survivor, and champion for change. Finding Solid Footing is essential reading for sepsis survivors and their loved ones, as well as for anyone seeking a better understanding of the profound impact of this under-recognized public health crisis." – **Thomas Heymann**, President and CEO, Sepsis Alliance

~

"Sepsis has been around as long as humans have had infections, maybe 2500 years. In the past, it was often fatal. Today, it is highly treatable if caught early. However, it still remains the #1 cause of death in most hospitals. Sepsis is truly a 'blanket of death, disability, and despair,' and Katy Grainger experienced all of this. In *Finding Solid Footing*, she shares her miraculous and vivid recovery from near death, through the entire progression of a minor infection to septic shock, amputations, survival, and recovery. She not only beat the odds of dying, but she also became a new person of vigor, faith, and purpose. She is an inspiring role model for anyone affected by this devastating syndrome. This book is a road map for anyone who feels they have lost their physical, emotional, and entire being, for whatever reason!" – **Carl Flatley**, DDS, MSD, Founder of Sepsis Alliance

~

"This book feels like being welcomed into Katy's living room, settling into a soft chair, and listening to someone who has lived through the unthinkable yet somehow grown brighter because of it. Katy doesn't just tell you what happened - she lets you feel the wobble of coming home after sepsis, the strangeness of meeting a body that no longer matches memory, and the quiet courage it takes to keep choosing life when everything feels unfamiliar. This isn't just a story about surviving sepsis or losing limbs. It's about becoming someone new without losing who you were. It's about finding radiance in places you never expected. And reading it feels like a privilege." – **Leslie Green**, MA, MA, MA, MA, MSW, Ed.S, Director Patient Advocacy & Education, Hanger Clinic

~

"Katy Grainger has a rare gift: she walks into a room, opens her heart, and makes every person in it feel seen. I've had the privilege of sharing a stage with her, and her story doesn't just move people - it stays with them. In my work on antimicrobial resistance, I spend a great deal of time thinking about what's at stake when infections can no longer be treated. *Finding Solid Footing* puts a profoundly human face on that reality. Katy's encounter with a drug-resistant infection - and everything that followed - is a powerful reminder that behind every policy discussion, there is a person fighting their way back from the unimaginable. Her courage in telling that story, with such honesty and grace, is a gift to anyone who has ever had to find solid footing after the ground gave way." – **Emily Wheeler**, Vice President of Infectious Disease Policy, Biotechnology Innovation Organization (BIO)

~

"As one of Katy's rehabilitation physicians, I witnessed firsthand the gravity of what she and her family faced. Sepsis is devastating, and the physical toll of limb loss alone is immense, let alone the emotional toll of facing a near-death experience and resulting lifelong disability. Yet what struck me most was how Katy and those around her met that sudden reality with remarkable courage and resilience from the very beginning. Katy's story captures something rarely conveyed in medical textbooks: recovery doesn't happen to one person in isolation. She tells her story not only from her own perspective, but through the experiences of her husband, children, friends, and caregivers. *Finding Solid Footing* is an honest and inspiring portrait of rehabilitation as a shared journey, which reflects the true spirit of team-based care. For anyone touched by serious illness, disability, or the experience of caring for someone through trauma or medical crisis, this book is an inspiring read." – **Janna L. Friedly**, MD, MPH, Professor and Chair, UW Medicine, Editor in Chief, *PM&R*

~

"I cannot remember the last time a book moved me to tears as often as *Finding Solid Footing*. In this evocative and courageous telling of her journey through suffering and into wholeness, Katy Grainger speaks the universal language of the soul. With breathtaking vulnerability and unflinching honesty, she invites us behind the curtain and lights a path for anyone walking through visible or invisible pain. Katy reminds us that suffering does not discriminate - and neither does hope. Her story is a profound testament that the way *out* is indeed *through*, and that grace often meets us first in our deepest fractures. This book is more than a memoir. It is a lifeline - a powerful invitation to reclaim our true identity, trust the healing process, and become beacons of hope for others. *Finding Solid Footing* has the potential not only to transform lives, but to save them." – **Morgan Snyder**, Author of *Becoming a King*

~

"I've known Katy from before this happened, and to watch how she navigated something she never chose was both impressive and deeply inspiring. Her honesty reveals a real depth of strength and humanity - nothing polished, just true. And that's what stays with you." – **Gabby Reece**, Host of The Gabby Reece Show, and Advocate for Health at Every Age

"A breathtakingly honest and deeply moving story of what it means to thrive beyond tragedy. I met Katy at a snowboarding event with my organization, Adaptive Action Sports, and was instantly struck by how closely her journey mirrors my own. We both faced septic shock and limb loss, and found our way forward. *Finding Solid Footing* is a powerful reminder that our spirit is never broken, even when our bodies are changed, and that hope and possibility are always within reach." – **Amy Purdy**, Keynote Speaker, NY Times Bestseller, and 3x Paralympic Medalist

"Katy Grainger is a dynamic voice of strength and perspective in both the sepsis and limb loss communities. Her story, as told in *Finding Solid Footing*, is raw, powerful, and deeply human. This is the kind of book that doesn't just inspire you, it changes the way you see your own life." – **Rick Bontkowski**, Host of The AMP'D UP211 Podcast

"Perhaps what's most remarkable about this book is what you won't find in it: a victim. It's simply astonishing the fortitude and can-do ethos Katy has embodied throughout this transformative experience. It is impossible to overstate the amount of good she has done not just for the sepsis survivor and amputee communities, but for anyone suffering a medical nightmare and anyone caring for them. She has turned a personal crisis into an opportunity for progress, healing, and wholeness for herself and so many others. That is the triumph of inner strength that leaps off every page, and the spirit of purpose that beams from Katy if you are fortunate enough to know her." – **Ashley Shearer**, LCSW, CSAC, Vice President, Care Coordination, Patient Flow, Geriatrics & Inpatient Rehabilitation, The Queen's Medical Center

~

"*Finding Solid Footing* is a powerful and deeply human account of resilience in its truest form. Having spent my career working with individuals navigating limb loss, I understand both the physical and emotional complexity of that journey - but Katy Grainger's story brings a rare level of honesty, courage, and clarity. Her journey resonates far beyond the limb loss community, offering hope and encouragement to anyone facing unexpected hardship. This book is more than a story - it is a testament to the resilience of the human spirit, the power of faith, and the courage it takes to reclaim life after profound loss." –**Jay Martin**, CP, FAAOP, CEO & Founder, Slingshot Bionics

~

"If you're a doctor or nurse who cares for patients with sepsis, you must read this book. If you have survived an episode of sepsis, you must read this book. If someone you love had sepsis, you must read this book. If you might ever have sepsis - and that means all of us - you must read this book. Once I started, it was hard to put down. I thank Katy for helping me to understand even better how my patients experience the nightmare. And how they can regain themselves and even surpass themselves with the support of the people who love them." – **Steven Q. Simpson**, MD, Professor of Medicine, University of Kansas

~

"My big takeaway from Katy Grainger's story of resilience is that none of us stands alone. We can only find solid footing through our connections to each other. [...] Without a rich community around us, Grainger tells us, none of us is complete. But when we weave ourselves into the tapestry that surrounds us, we become whole - no matter what losses we're called to endure along the way." –**Larry Borowsky**, Amplitude magazine

~

"Katy Grainger's story stays with you - deeply and personally. Having spent decades in critical care, bearing witness to the profound physiologic collapse and often unimaginable suffering that sepsis can bring, I read her story through a very real and clinical lens. I have seen how quickly this disease strips patients of control, stability, and sometimes hope. And yet, this is exactly why Katy's story is so powerful. She captures not only the brutality of critical illness, but something we as clinicians also quietly witness at the bedside - the extraordinary resilience of the human spirit. Katy writes with honesty, warmth, and clarity, allowing readers to feel the depth of her struggle while also showing what is possible on the other side. *Finding Solid Footing* is more than a memoir - it is a guide, a companion through some of life's most difficult terrain." – **Barbara McLean** MN RN CCNS-BC NP-BC CCRN FCCM MCCM, Critical Care Program Specialist, Grady Health Systems

~

"*Finding Solid Footing* is a moving memoir of survival and resilience, chronicling Katy Grainger's journey through sepsis, amputation, and recovery with raw honesty and hope. It's a powerful reminder of the strength of the human spirit, the importance of advocacy, and the healing power of community and family. The book traces how Katy refuses to let catastrophe be the end of the story, instead shaping it into a calling rooted in advocacy, education, and presence for others walking similar paths." – **Rosemary Grant** BSN, RN, CPHQ, CPPS, Director, Clinical Excellence, Washington State Hospital Association

~

"*Finding Solid Footing* is a profoundly moving testament to the resilience of the human spirit. Chronicling Katy Grainger's harrowing battle with sudden septic shock and the resulting amputations, this memoir is an unforgettable story of thriving beyond unimaginable tragedy. Grainger writes with raw honesty about her darkest moments and her most agonizing choices, but ultimately delivers a powerful message of hope, the life-saving impact of a loving community, and the fierce courage required to reclaim a joyful life." – **Kathleen M. Vollman** MSN, RN, CCNS, FCCM, FCNS, FAAN, Clinical Nurse Specialist/Consultant, Advancing Nursing, LLC

~

"Katy writes with an honesty that is both vulnerable and fierce at the same time. The way she frames her process of surrender to the brutal devastation of sepsis is held together by her prophetic words, 'the only way out was through.' Katy's is a story of a phoenix rising from the ashes. Not just rising, but thriving and recreating a life she never imagined. Katy's truthful storytelling invites an onramp for all to consider the tiny steps our lives might require, leading us to deeper places of faith, relationship, opportunity, passion, and purpose." – **Rev. Paul Barrett**, Pastor and Head of Staff, St. Peter's by the Sea Presbyterian Church

~

"This is an extraordinary memoir that turns pain and tragedy into power. Katy doesn't just survive - she teaches us how to live again after the unthinkable happens. Katy's story is a testament to resilience and the healing power of community. Her honesty and courage will inspire anyone facing life's hardest challenges. Her story reminds us that even in loss, we can find purpose." – **Pat Posa**, RN, BSN, MSA, CCRN, FAAN, Quality and Safety Manager, Hospital Safety Consortium (HMS) Sepsis, University of Michigan

~

"Katy is the kind of friend you meet and never want to let go of - and yet, we almost lost her. In these pages, she shares a story marked by unimaginable loss and fierce resilience, inviting us into her vulnerability and revealing a depth of courage and aliveness that calls us to examine our own lives with the same honesty." – **Lindsay Murphy**, Associate Pastor, Mercer Island Presbyterian Church

FOR MY FAMILY

This is my love letter to you

CONTENTS

PROLOGUE

"I can't go back to yesterday because I was a different person then."

– *Alice in Wonderland* by Lewis Carroll

Floored

I wake up on the cold, hard floor in complete darkness. My eyes blink as I strain to see where I am.

My knees and feet are aching. A sharp pain is emanating from my right ankle. My head feels like it's been hit by something hard.

The air around me is warm and humid, but I'm shivering.

How long have I been lying here?

I have no idea where I am or what's happened.

Where's the Mad Hatter? What happened to Belle? We were just having tea…

The room blurs and fades to black.

A rooster crows in the distance. I open my eyes again. I try to remember.

That's right, I'm on the floor. But why?

I call out for my husband, Scott, expecting him to be nearby. There's no response.

Am I still in California? Why is there a rooster in my hotel room?

I try to lift my head, despite the dizziness and the painful, rhythmic throbbing, synchronized with my racing heart.

In the dim light, a bed comes into focus across the room. With a sense of relief, I recognize the blue-and-white comforter as my own.

This is my room in Hanalei!

I try to move but quickly collapse back into a shivering heap of pain and confusion. I call out for Scott again. Still no answer.

Wasn't I just with my girls in California?

I was having tea with my twenty-year-old daughter Jordan on a child-sized table by the Teacup ride at Disneyland. The Mad Hatter was there, and Belle from *Beauty and the Beast.* The Mad Hatter poured imaginary tea while Belle talked about her love of reading. My daughter, who has always loved to read, was lit up like a six-year-old meeting her childhood hero.

But I'm not in Disneyland now. Am I?

I look around the bedroom, searching for clues.

How did I get here? What's happening?!

The floor is so cold. I want to get up, but even the slightest attempt to lift my body hurts.

Something's wrong! I need help!

I'm too confused and exhausted to know what to do.

I'll just close my eyes for a minute.

I wake up again, on the floor next to my bed. The room is not as dark now, but I'm still so cold.

How long was I asleep? How did I get over here?

My knees feel bruised and raw. The soft mattress, pillows, and welcoming blankets seem out of reach above me.

If I can just get into my bed, everything will be okay…

I shiver in the Hawaiian heat as I struggle to hoist my broken body onto my bed, exhaustion numbing the pain coursing through me.

I drift off to sleep, unaware or unconcerned that I may never wake up again.

INTRODUCTION

"You are never too old to set another goal, or to dream a new dream."

– C. S. Lewis

A Story to Tell

"You have a story to tell," she told me. I knew she wasn't wrong.

I'd been so anxious about this meeting. Although I was excited to be getting out of my house to meet with close friends, the occasion was overshadowed by my fear of running into people I knew who may not have heard about my life-threatening battle with sepsis and the amputations that followed. I was terrified I would see someone who wasn't adequately prepared to confront the changes in my body. I didn't want to witness their initial reaction of shock, fear, or pity. I knew I couldn't handle that.

How can I comfort someone else over what happened to me and my body? I can barely cope with my own emotions.

I was even nervous about seeing my good friend Kathryn, who knew my whole story but hadn't met up with me since I'd gotten sick. She had seen photos of me on Facebook after my surgeries, but the last time we met in person, I was healthy and fit.

How will she react to seeing me in a wheelchair, missing my feet, lower legs, and seven fingertips?

Using the same muscles I had used as a child to lift myself onto the beam in gymnastics, I lifted my body out of the car and into the waiting wheelchair. Todd, my nurse-turned-best-friend, held the wheelchair firmly against the car while I got situated. He carefully covered my legs with a blanket to obscure the empty space where feet should be. He protectively placed his hand on my shoulder as he backed my chair out from behind the car door, up the wheelchair ramp, and into the restaurant.

As Todd awkwardly maneuvered my wheelchair through the restaurant doors, we saw Kathryn's beautiful face beaming at me from the nearest table. She had thoughtfully requested an open space for my wheelchair to make my entrance as smooth as possible. Kathryn didn't look down at my body. She just kept looking into my eyes with that huge, welcoming smile of hers.

This was the look I had seen on the faces of all the friends who had visited me over the prior weeks; a look that told me, "You're so much more than your fingertips. You're so much more than your lower legs. You are Katy, the same woman we've always known. You're my friend and confidante, and that hasn't changed. I'm so happy to see you. I'm so glad you're still here."

Even when the voice in my head told me otherwise, this look from my friends and family reminded me daily that I was still me.

Once we'd settled in, Kathryn extended her invitation, "Please be my guest at a writing workshop I'm hosting at my home in a few months. You have a *big* story to tell."

She had a valid point. I'd been telling my story almost daily to friends and family who visited or called to check in on me. I'd grown accustomed to seeing the shock on their faces as they heard horrific, almost unbelievable events of the past few months. I knew I had experienced something extraordinary, but my family and I were still in the trenches, slogging through the most difficult time of our lives. To everyone I encountered along the way, though, ours was a story of survival… a story of hope, endurance, and overcoming loss. While I was sharing my tragedy, they were hearing an inspirational story.

When Kathryn went on to explain that the writing instructor for this workshop was Beth Bornstein Dunnington, I was intrigued. I had heard good things about Beth's talent for helping women of all ages find their voices and share their stories in her "Big Island Writers' Workshop." But writing a book? That still felt light years ahead of where I was that day.

I was still so overwhelmed by all that happened and the healing process that had overtaken my life. Besides, I felt like it was pure luck that I had survived, which wasn't worthy of a book. *Lucky Me*, by Katy Grainger, wasn't something even I would read, let alone expect strangers to read.

Still, a seed was planted that day. This was the first of many seeds planted along the way that would bring me to the happiness, success, and fulfillment I'm finally experiencing today. With the help of supporters like Kathryn, Beth – whose writers' workshops gave birth to a number of the chapters written in this book – and Adrienne, my indispensable editor and "memoir midwife," those seeds have grown into the book you hold in your hands today.

A Book to Write

"We don't have to do it all alone. We were never meant to."

– Brené Brown

As time went on, and more and more people chimed in on the "You need to write a book" chorus, I started to listen.

I listened when they told me I needed to educate others about the signs and symptoms of sepsis, and the importance of knowing when to get medical help.

I listened when they urged me to speak up about the importance of taking a person with you to the emergency room in case you can't speak for yourself, and to help doctors understand the symptoms that are unusual for you, so you're not misdiagnosed or dismissed.

I listened when they encouraged me to share what it was like to wake up in the ICU with extreme delirium, and to slog through months of painful recovery, in the hospital and at home. I listened when they told me to share what I'd learned about both the mental and physical health toll that medical trauma can have on a patient and their caregivers, and offer tips for living with and recovering from these complications.

I was sharing all of this information with my friends, and they kept telling me more people needed to hear it. As I became stronger, I began to believe that.

Now, six years after Kathryn's invitation to join Beth Bornstein Dunnington's writing workshop, where I continue to mine for stories to this day, my sepsis experience and disability are no longer the focus of my time, and my life has returned to an altered version of the life I knew before. But the lessons I've learned along the way have been invaluable and expanded my world in ways I never could have imagined.

I have come to appreciate all the experiences that shaped my life into what it is today.

We constantly experience opportunities for change, for better or worse. We can't control what happens to us, only how we handle it. The choice is ours to make. We grow, or we choose not to grow. We adapt, or we don't. The quality of our life after tragedy, illness, or loss reflects our response, not the event itself.

The work doesn't need to be hard, and it doesn't need to be continual. There can and will be steps forward and steps back. There can and will be good days and bad days. We just need to keep moving forward at our own pace.

As the wise Dory reminds us in the Disney/Pixar film *Finding Nemo*, "Just keep swimming!"

As I have faced my recovery, walking forward one day and falling back another, I have slowly but surely reclaimed my life. Accepting that some days would be complete failures helped me wake up the next day and start fresh.

My goal every week is for my good days to outnumber my bad days, and for my steps forward to outpace my steps backward. That's how I've approached my whole recovery, and it's paid off in spades.

As you read through my story, I invite you to remember that it isn't mine alone. I didn't survive alone or recover alone. I didn't learn to share my stories alone or write and publish a book alone. This is one of the greatest lessons of my journey: we are only as alone as we choose to be, and there's never a good enough reason to struggle in silence.

Speak up. Ask for the support you deserve. With help, we can all do so much more than we ever imagined.

Above all, don't be afraid to get your story out there. You never know who may need it.

CHAPTER 1

INTO THE EMPTY NEST

"There are only three answers to a prayer: 'yes,' 'not yet,' and 'I have something else in mind for you.' Man's great challenge is trusting 'not yet" or 'something else.' "

– Elsa Dutton, *1923*, Season 1, Episode 3

Greece, September 14, 2017

My eyes filled with tears as I looked down at my hands, dribbling red, sticky droplets onto the weathered white stones.

My life as I know it is gone. What comes next?

The invitation to come on this Greek Odyssey could not have come at a more poignant time. My youngest daughter had just flown the nest, heading off to the mainland for college and leaving me behind in Hawaii to grapple with my identity.

I had spent two decades raising my two beautiful girls, revolving my life around theirs, staying constantly prepared to meet their every need, and looking for every opportunity to empower them to thrive on their own. Now that they were doing just that, I found myself wondering, *Who am I without them?*

My first instinct was to jump forward in time, praying they would become mothers in a few years and that I could have a new purpose in helping to raise and impart wisdom to my grandchildren. That would be easy for me; caring for children was a job I knew well. But in my heart, I knew I needed to find purpose within myself, beyond the roles I played for others.

Don't get me wrong, I found plenty of ways to fill my time: making weekly snacks and sandwiches for a local after-school program; spending time with my husband and friends; doing yoga, biking, and swimming; entertaining mainland friends, and showing them my beloved Kauai. But I was still searching for a central focus to give my life the same fulfillment, purpose, and meaning I'd enjoyed while raising my kids.

I prayed. I meditated. I set the intention to find a new calling. I focused on strengthening my body and mind with healthy food and exercise, stimulation from books and podcasts, and time with friends and my husband. I knew I couldn't force my calling to declare itself, but I could prepare myself to recognize when it was revealed.

So when Jeanette, a friend from Hanalei, invited me to join her on a women's trip to Greece aimed at "connecting to the goddess within," it felt like an answer to my prayers, or at least an opportunity to find my own answers. I said yes immediately.

Surrounded by fellow/sister seekers, I would discover my goddess self and what she had in store for the remainder of my life. Which goddess would be revealed as I peeled away the roles I had played for others – daughter, wife, mother? Was I Artemis, Aphrodite, or maybe even Hera?

In the course of the journey, I came to realize I didn't have to choose: every woman embodies the traits and power of every goddess. As we move through our lives, we connect with different stories and call upon various abilities at different times.

For example, when I first learned Greek Mythology in school, I resonated with the story of Persephone, daughter of the harvest goddess Demeter. I felt for the beautiful teen who was just minding her own business, picking flowers by the ocean, when her uncle Hades abducted her and dragged her down to the underworld.

I could relate to her anguish when, even after returning to Earth and reuniting with her mother, she realized she'd been tricked into eating pomegranate seeds, the food of the underworld, thereby signing herself up to live a third of every year in Hades' realm as long as she lived. How could she have known that just by consuming that small amount of fruit, she was not only denying herself time on Earth but also denying her mother precious time with her only daughter?

Yet, years later, when I heard the story again in Greece, standing outside the Nekromantheon near Ephyra, the very spot where she's said to have been taken into the underworld, it wasn't Persephone I related to, but her mother, Demeter. I pictured myself in ragged, once-green robes, inconsolable, relentlessly searching every corner of the Earth for my beloved daughter with my magical torch, wondering if I would ever find her and who I would be without her.

That magical torch was gifted to Demeter by the Titan Hecate, who would later use her special powers to rescue Persephone from the underworld. Triple goddesses like Hecate embody the trinity of all of the phases in a woman's life: maiden (youth), mother (middle age), and crone, or wise woman (elder years). I had seen my daughters in the maiden Persephone and me in the mother Demeter. But in Hecate, I saw us all as one.

Hecate embodied the transitions I was struggling with: from the young maiden of my youth to the mother I had been for so many years, to the wise woman I was becoming. Confronted with the reality that my girls had left maidenhood and I was maturing from mother to crone, I came seeking clarity before these three goddesses, Persephone, Demeter, and Hecate.

What purpose did I have outside of my girls, my husband, and my family? What could my wisdom, experience, and passion do for this world in the last third of my life? What was the meaning of my life as a wise woman?

These questions led me to the Nekromantheon in Greece, to make my sacrificial offering. My hands dripped with that red, sticky juice as I tore open the pomegranate I'd carried with me to this powerful place. When I saw the insides teeming with shiny scarlet seeds, each carrying the possibility of new life, just as my body had once teemed with life in the form of my unborn daughters, my eyes filled with tears. Tears of grief for what was, but also tears of joy for what might be.

That day, I loosened my emotional grip on the young women to whom I had given birth and raised, and felt a sense of pride as I recognized they were becoming adults. I experienced renewed strength in my presence as a mother, realizing that my daughters and their children would always need and appreciate me in this role. This freed me to let go of my resistance and begin to accept my new identity as a wise woman. But who would I be in this role?

I prayed for guidance. I prayed for wisdom. I prayed for a purpose.

I had faith that my prayers would be answered. I left Greece with a sense of peace I hadn't felt in years.

How could I have known the purpose I prayed for would arrive a year later, in the form of a tragedy that would permanently alter my body and my life?

I was expecting a religious epiphany or "aha" moment. Instead, I got the miracle of survival and recovery – proof that the Lord does indeed work in mysterious ways.

It would be years before I recognized the tragedy of sepsis for what it was: an unexpected and messy answer to my prayers.

My new mission. My new calling. My new purpose.

But this story doesn't begin on an island in Greece. It starts on the island of Kauai, in Hawaii. And, as is so often the case, to get where we're going, we first need to take a step back. A decade back, to be exact, to another island altogether.

Mercer Island, Washington, 2008

Blame it on the iPhone

It's no coincidence that the decision my husband, Scott, and I made to take a year-long break from living on Mercer Island coincided with the release of the first iPhone. This handheld device would connect every user to the internet from anywhere, including playgrounds, automobiles, and school buses. We knew it wouldn't be long before internet-connected phones became the norm and everyone would have a computer in their pocket. We were anxious about how quickly the world was changing, especially for our kids.

We wanted to take a year away from the Seattle area to offer our girls the chance to experience lives more like the ones we'd enjoyed growing up in Spokane in the 70's: less pressure and stress, and more time enjoying the outdoors and the company of friends and family.

We considered adventures like renting an RV to road-trip across the United States or traveling to another country to immerse ourselves in a new culture. But we wanted this time away to feel less like a new job and more like a break for Scott and me, so we opted for something simpler and closer to home: a year on the Northshore of Kauai, Hawaii, in a little surfing town we'd enjoyed visiting on vacation.

After nearly 25 years in the Seattle area, we longed for warmer weather, longer winter days, more time in nature, and a break from the rat race of city life. Hanalei offered us the small-town experience and close-knit community we'd been craving. It had small schools that encouraged experiential learning and individualism, along with immersion in nature and the community. We rented our Mercer Island home to friends, then we signed the girls up for school on Kauai and took the leap.

Hanalei, Hawaii

Kauai is known as the Garden Island for good reason. As the oldest of the Hawaiian islands, it's had the most time to grow a thick layer of diverse vegetation over its dramatic landscape. The iconic mountains are thickly forested and flowing with magnificent waterfalls. The area feels like a tropical jungle, with taro fields reaching deep into the valley, tall buffalo grass growing in the open spaces, and green lawns and tropical gardens around the homes. Coconut trees grow wild along the beaches, across open spaces, and in many yards. There are endangered birds that breed there and wild chickens everywhere. Every home has a few resident geckos that break the silence with their little chirping "laughs."

Hanalei is a small surfing town, nestled in a luscious valley between three gorgeous mountains and the Pacific Ocean. The town consists of taro farms, small shops and restaurants, an elementary school, a rural post office, and several churches. The residents include local families, vacationers, and transplants like us, seeking the experience of a simpler time.

The environment is inviting on both sunny days and during the warm showers that are a hallmark of life in Hanalei. Once or twice every winter, it rains so hard that the Hanalei bridge closes due to rising flood waters, resulting in school closures we lovingly refer to as "Hawaiian snow days."

When we first moved there, we were told that Hawaii chooses the people she allows to stay. We prayed she would welcome our family and let us call her our home. She did.

We were embraced by the community, initially through a dear friend who had lived his whole life in Hanalei, and through our daughters' soccer teams. Soccer was a big part of our lives in Mercer Island, and we were thrilled to find competitive teams on Kauai. Both girls excelled at soccer and Scott loved coaching, so we fit in nicely with the other parents and kids. We used this as an opportunity to make our first friends.

Just as we'd hoped, life in Hanalei was more like the life we'd known as kids. Classes were small and pressure was low. Kids played outside until dusk and came inside to do homework and have dinner. We didn't even own a television that first year because our days were so full, enjoying new friends and life near the ocean.

Scott and I can't recall who was the first to suggest that we remain in Hawaii permanently. We just agreed on it one day and didn't look back. After all, our prayers had been answered. Hawaii had invited us to stay. Why would we ever leave?

CHAPTER 2

MISTAKES WERE MADE

"The body never lies."

– Martha Graham

Friday Afternoon, September 14, 2018 (10 years later)

It was a tiny bump. No bigger than a mosquito bite. So minuscule, so innocuous.

How could I have known that something so small could tear such a massive hole in my life?

I first noticed it on the flight back to Kauai from California, where I'd just spent two weeks visiting my daughters. There it was, this little bump on my thumb. It was the color of a fresh bruise, with a small, oozing break in the skin.

Even though it was tiny, something about it gave me pause. Maybe it was the color. Maybe it was the fluid oozing from it. Maybe it was pure intuition. Whatever it was, it led me to a walk-in medical clinic before heading to our secluded North Shore home.

I wanted to be extra sure everything was okay since it was a Friday, and I knew the only clinic within reasonable driving distance of my home would be closed over the weekend. Scott was in Idaho on a fly-fishing trip, so if things went sideways, I'd be on my own. When you live in the tropics, things like MRSA and other drug-resistant bacteria can spread quickly without antibiotics to keep them in check. Better safe than sorry, I figured.

At the clinic, they took my vital signs, including blood pressure, heart rate, breathing rate, temperature, and blood oxygen level. They were all normal; no indication of illness. So far, so good.

My doctor took a swab of the infection on my thumb to identify the cause, but warned me it would take a few days to get results. In the meantime, he gave me a prescription-strength topical antibiotic ointment and prescribed oral antibiotics, which he said I should take if the bump didn't improve by the next morning.

The nurse handed me a packet of information that included notes from my appointment, symptoms, diagnosis, and a recommendation to "Please return to the clinic in three days if not better. Call or return to the clinic sooner if your condition worsens, or if you have any concerns."

And with that, they sent me on my way.

When it Rains, it Pours

As I waited for my turn to cross the one-lane bridge into Hanalei, I couldn't help but smile. I was remembering the tears of joy that had poured down my face the day I'd come down this same hill, knowing this magical place was now my home. Jason Mraz's "I'm Yours" was blasting on the stereo as I'd made the hairpin turn and been treated to this outrageous view of the three iconic mountains: Hihimanu, Namolokama, and Mamalahoa. They were decked out in every shade of green with the fertile Hanalei Valley stretching out to the majestic waves of Hanalei Bay.

I couldn't believe we were finally making this dream come true!

After driving a half mile along the Hanalei River, the main strip of town came into view and another memory surfaced. In April, half a year earlier, the road I was driving on had been submerged in muddy water from the most destructive flood in recorded Hanalei history.

I thought back to those floods as I headed to the home that had once been my sanctuary, but which no longer felt as safe as it had before the big storm. Though it wasn't a hurricane, rain fell unabated for three days, unleashing 50 inches of rain in 24 hours. It was both horrifying and awe-inspiring: intense, relentless, and deafeningly loud at times. The north shore of Kauai was transformed into temporary wetlands as water quickly backed up storm drains, overflowing pools and ponds. It seeped into anything at ground level, including septic tanks and cesspools, as well as most homes in the valley.

In the middle of the night on April 14, 2018, I was in our backyard helping Scott push rainwater away from our house with a wide push broom when movement in my peripheral vision caught my eye. Turning my head, I saw something incomprehensible: a two-foot wave of muddy water rushing into our yard from the direction of the mountains.

The ankle-deep water I'd been wading through was suddenly up to my knees. I ran inside with Scott as debris-filled floodwater gushed in behind us. I was trying to make sense of what had just happened as I stood on our stairs, watching the opaque brown water swallow our bottom three steps.

We lived in the middle of the valley, about a mile from each of the surrounding rivers, so flooding at our house seemed inconceivable. I was dumbfounded by what I was witnessing. I knew it wasn't a tsunami, because I had seen with my own eyes that it came from the opposite direction of the ocean.

Scott and I walked upstairs, drenched and speechless. We looked out our windows, watching the lightning flashes light up the valley and reveal dark water in every direction, as far as we could see.

We later learned that the excessive rainfall on the mountains surrounding our valley had caused a wall of water to sweep through town like a reverse tsunami, heading to the sea. The rivers on either side of our town flooded more than at any time in recorded history, causing standing water across town up to eight feet deep in places, and millions of dollars in damage.

We worked with the community to help others and were blessed to have a Christian mission group come to our home to help us remove all the saturated drywall, which had become a haven for black mold and other health-threatening microbes. We spent months cleaning our yard and repairing the ground floor of our house; we met regularly with friends to swap stories of the big storm.

As I drove through town with that odd infection on my thumb, I couldn't help but wonder if bacteria left behind by that flood had caused it.

If so, this could be a real problem.

When the local grocery store came into view, it occurred to me that I might not have a thermometer at home. Even though I was exhausted and anxious to get home, I stopped and bought one.

If the infection on my thumb is making me sick, I'll get a fever. That'll be my cue that the antibiotics aren't working and I need urgent medical attention.

I was wrong. Dead wrong.

My belief that I needed a fever to be deathly ill was a false one. One that nearly cost me my life.

Home, Sweet Home

As I pulled our truck onto the grass in front of our tucked-away home, I was relieved and unsettled at the same time. With no neighbors closer than a quarter mile away, it was both an ideal retreat from the outside world and an isolated spot where no one would hear me call for help if something went wrong.

My footsteps echoed through the large, open-plan house as I entered, armed with my new thermometer and antibiotics. I locked the door behind me, checked to make sure the sliding glass door to the backyard was locked, and headed upstairs to the kitchen.

I had scheduled my trip home on Friday so I could make it to the birthday party of one of my best friends. But once I had everything unloaded and climbed the second flight of stairs to my bedroom, I was utterly wiped out. I called my friend Tiffany, who had planned the party, and told her I was too exhausted from traveling to drive back up to Princeville. She was understanding and encouraged me to rest.

Just before I hung up, though, intuition struck. I remembered a pact I had made with my girls that we would always ask a friend or family member to check on us whenever we were sick.

We'd made that pact three years earlier when Julia, a close friend of my daughter Dani's, had become critically ill from a strep throat infection and nearly died because she was alone in her dorm when it happened. She ended up in the ICU in septic shock just 24 hours after visiting Health Services at her college. She spent over a month in the hospital, suffered a loss of circulation to her feet, and ended up having one of her lower legs amputated.

The only reason Julia survived was that her roommate happened to come home and find her unconscious in her bed. When she had difficulty waking Julia up and saw that her skin was ashen and her lips tinged blue, she called an ambulance.

My family and I were stunned by the news of her hospitalization and amputation. This vibrant young woman, who is like family to us, was suddenly an amputee. She would likely have died had her roommate not checked in on her when she did. I had never heard of such a thing happening; it seemed impossible that something as simple as strep throat, which she'd had many times before, could lead to this kind of life-altering health crisis, especially in someone so healthy.

Until then, I had only heard the word sepsis in medical dramas. I had no idea how common it was in the real world or how quickly it could destroy or permanently alter a life. And despite what happened to Julia, I had never learned the symptoms.

Fortunately, Julia recovered and went on to thrive, but her experience led my family to make this pact that we would never be sick alone without making sure someone was checking on us.

Thanks to the sudden intrusion of that terrible memory, and despite feeling a bit silly, I forced myself to explain my situation to Tiffany. I told her about the infection and Scott being out of town, and asked her to do me a favor: could she please set an alarm on her phone to call me in the morning, just to make sure everything was okay?

She happily agreed. With that safety net in place, I relaxed and settled in for a peaceful weekend at home.

An Unexpected Danger

Looking out at the stunning view of the mountains as the sky began to dim that evening, my eyes were drawn to a tall, dark shape moving through the trees in my backyard. My stomach tightened. My pulse quickened. Was it an intruder? A pig hunter? If I were in danger, who would I call who could get there in time to help?

I heard our dogs, Olive and Buddy, sound the bark alarm as I strained to make out the dark shape lurking in the thick tropical foliage. But the harder I stared, the more it seemed to disappear into the shadows, until finally I couldn't see anything but darkness. No movement, no figure, no barking. Just the usual croaking of bullfrogs and swaying of palm fronds. I felt unsettled.

A little while later, I looked for the information packet I'd been handed on my way out of the clinic and realized I'd left it on my passenger seat. I was too tired and anxious to go outside to get it, so I did my best to recall what symptoms I'd been told would alert me to take the oral antibiotics. I was still under the false impression that a fever would let me know if I was getting sick.

I texted Scott a photo of my hand showing the bump on my thumb, and let him know I had seen a doctor and asked a friend to check in on me so he wouldn't worry. Looking back, I think my gut was telling me the infection might be significant, even though the photo looked like little more than a bruise-colored mosquito bite.

My stomach wasn't feeling quite right, which I blamed on a combination of traveling and anxiety, so I skipped dinner and took a relaxing bath. I lit scented candles and placed them around a bathtub of sudsy water infused with lavender bath salts. I wanted to make the best of this time alone while Scott was out of town.

As the water around me cooled, I looked out over our peaceful koi pond and talked on the phone with one of my best friends back in Seattle, letting her know I was home safe from my travels. Just for fun, I sent her a picture of my lower legs and feet in the tub, bragging about my plans for my special week of relaxation and pampering while Scott was away.

Before bed, I took my temperature. It was normal.

Nothing to worry about.

I crawled under the covers just after sunset and pulled them tight around my neck as I had as a little girl to feel safe in my bed. I slept through the night, blissfully unaware that the two photos I had just texted to Scott and Kamma would be the last photos ever taken of my healthy hands and feet.

CHAPTER 3

FALLING DOWN THE RABBIT HOLE

"The little girl just could not sleep, because her thoughts were way too deep, her mind had gone out for a stroll and fallen down the rabbit hole."

– Lewis Carroll, *Alice in Wonderland*

Saturday Morning, September 15, 2018

I woke up later than usual, having slept through the crowing Hanalei roosters that usually awakened me. I looked forward to a lazy day of resting and unwinding from my travels, maybe doing some laundry and unpacking my bags.

The infection on my thumb had grown larger overnight, changing from a deep scarlet pink to an ominous dark purple. So again, I took my temperature. Still no fever. In fact, my temperature registered a bit low. I assumed I hadn't left the thermometer in my mouth long enough, but I figured I was fine.

Truthfully, I don't remember much beyond this point because I was so much sicker than I realized. I pieced together the following time-line from photos and text exchanges on my phone.

At 7:15 a.m., I took a picture of my thumb next to a ruler, slick and shiny with antibiotic ointment, to show the size of the infection. It looked like a blood blister with an opaque covering, as if the infection was deep beneath all the layers of my skin. I probably took the photo to show the progression to Scott, or a doctor if needed.

An hour later, I called Tiffany and told her not to worry about checking in on me again; the antibiotics would take care of the infection, and I would call her if anything changed. I'm sure that at this point, both of us thought I was going to be just fine.

9:06 a.m. - Katy - text to Scott:

> I'm feeling ok. Thought I was getting a fever last night. Going back to sleep. Dogs are great. Love you! 🩶

No mention of the color change in my wound or that I had just told Tiffany there was no need to check in on me again. I wonder what made me think I was getting a fever the night before?

After a shower, I decided to crawl back into the comfort of my bed and sleep a little longer. After all, I was in vacation mode. I had the house to myself since Scott was gone for at least another week, and I could relax in bed for as long as I wanted. I figured I just needed a little extra rest.

My friends texted, inviting me to meet them at the Hanalei Farmers Market, which is within easy walking distance of my house. I told them I was tired and was going to stay home for the day to relax. They offered to bring me lunch, but I assured them I had lots of food and would be fine.

It seems like I spent most of the next 24 hours in bed. During that time, I texted back and forth with many of my mainland friends and family, thanking them for our time together on my trip and letting them know I had arrived safely back on Kauai. I was also checking in on a few friends I hadn't had a chance to see while I was in Seattle. I never mentioned feeling sick or overly tired.

2:00 p.m. - Text to Scott:

> still hanging in there. Took the oral antibiotic. Because my thumb infection keeps growing. It's disgusting. How the heck did I get this?! I'll send a pic. I've never had anything like this. I knew immediately it was staph. 💕

I can tell by the wording and punctuation that I was using voice-to-text, which I only used when extremely tired or not feeling well.[1]

We texted a bit more, talking about his trip and plans. I seem coherent and in good spirits.

2:11 p.m. - Text to Scott:

> "I'm falling asleep. I will text you when I wake up. All is good. No fever. 😌🩶

Later in the day, we talked on the phone. I told him I had thrown up, but minimized that symptom by attributing it to having taken an antibiotic on an empty stomach.

Looking back, it's obvious I was dismissing multiple cues that I was getting sick from the infection because of my mistaken belief that all I needed to monitor was my temperature. The vomiting, excessive sleeping, and worsening infection were all concerning symptoms, but I was explaining them away.

Even my rationalizations held clues: the fact that I said I took an antibiotic without any food in my system was an indication that I was neither eating well nor thinking clearly. I'd been very sick before from taking medications on an empty stomach, so I knew better.

Infection, vomiting, and mental decline are all symptoms of sepsis. Had I known this, I would have been watching my symptoms more closely and called someone to be with me, just in case I got sicker.

---

1. When I mentioned "staph," I was referring to MRSA, a drug-resistant form of staphylococcus aureus, a bacteria found on human skin that can be difficult to treat without medical intervention.

Instead, I was doing the opposite: isolating myself and avoiding direct interactions.

I suspect I didn't want to bother anyone and was overconfident that I could take care of myself. As a mother, it was my role in the family to take care of everyone when they were sick. I hadn't considered that I would need help from others if I became ill.

Except for a quick phone call from Scott, all of my exchanges were by text. My sister-in-law Maren, who happens to be a doctor, called me. I responded with the automatic text you can select when talking on the phone: *"Sorry, I can't talk right now."* That must have been when I was talking to Scott, because I never got back to her. She wouldn't hear from me again until I was fighting for my life in the hospital and needed her medical advice.

A couple of my other friends said I didn't take their calls or respond to texts that afternoon. They would tell me this weeks later when I was trying to piece together my lost weekend.

Scott was the last correspondence I had that day, and I cut it short, saying I was tired.

The whole day, I was playing down everything to myself and the people I was texting.

"I'm okay," "I'm just tired," "It's no big deal," "I'll be fine."

I now understand the importance of talking with a person on the phone at the very least, or face-to-face whenever possible, when experiencing unusual symptoms. Had I insisted on having someone come by to check on me, this story would likely have had a much less dramatic ending.

Saturday Night

At some point during the night, I left my bed and walked up the three steps into my bathroom. My doctors later speculated that my blood pressure was low, causing me to pass out when I stood up from the toilet. Then I likely missed a step and fell onto the hardwood floor below.

I broke a small bone in my left foot, sprained my right ankle, and bruised and scraped my knee from the fall. I don't remember any of that happening. All I know is that, even after passing out and breaking a bone, I didn't call an ambulance or a friend for help. Instead, I apparently crawled across the floor where I passed out repeatedly on the way, then finally hoisted myself back into my bed and fell asleep.

It's clear, looking back, that I wasn't thinking straight, a strong indicator of going into septic shock. Had I not awoken the next morning and called for help, I could have died alone in my bed.

CHAPTER 4

LISTENING TO MY GUT

"Intuition is the whisper of the soul."

– Antoine de Saint-Exupéry

Sunday Morning, September 16, 2018

6:17 a.m. - Katy - text to Tiffany:

> "I'm really sick. Can you twk me to wilcox? I threw lup all afternoon and I can't pee. And I can barely walk. My balanc e I all messed Up. I have staph on my thumb and am worried it's spreading I've n v r b n to his sick"

Like so much of that weekend, I don't remember sending this text. But here's how I imagine it happening:

I picture myself sprawled on my bed – battered, bruised, broken bone in my left foot, sprained right ankle, sicker than I'd ever been – as dawn broke on Sunday. The sun, still tucked behind the mountains, lit up the sky, cueing the neighborhood roosters to issue their morning announcements with increasing confidence.

Was I floating in that unique mental space between asleep and awake when suddenly lucidity struck, and I realized how sick I was? Or did I somehow feel compelled to send out the only distress call I could manage, without fully understanding why?

Or maybe I had been waiting until dawn to reach out because it would be rude to wake a friend in the middle of the night. That sounds ridiculous, knowing now how sick I was then. But at the time, I didn't know.

Twice, in my younger years, I went to the hospital because of food poisoning. I couldn't stop vomiting. I got so weak I could no longer sit up from the bathroom floor to reach the toilet. Both times, I had a powerful instinct that something was really wrong and I needed urgent medical attention. And both times, it turned out to be a case of extreme dehydration.

At the hospital, I was given intravenous fluids and sent home within a few hours, feeling 90% back to my old self. It's a good bet that, as I descended into illness on Saturday night, I was framing this situation as just another case of acute dehydration, so calling for help in the middle of the night would have felt like overkill.

Little did I know that it was precisely the opposite.

Whatever my reasoning for sending Tiffany a text at that exact moment, lucky timing saved my life. Had it been any other morning, Tiffany wouldn't have received my text right away, and I might have died in my bed before she ever saw it.

6:18 a.m. - Tiffany - text to Katy:

> "Good morning. Just woke up. Yes I can take you. Do you want to go to urgent care first or Wilcox [hospital an hour away]?"

I later learned that Tiffany has a personal policy of never sleeping with her phone by her bed because she's a real estate agent and often gets calls at odd hours from people reaching out from different time zones. But the previous night, she just happened to fall asleep before taking her phone out of her room.

Though I have no memory of the first portion of this text exchange, I recall what happened next with chilling clarity.

I awoke with a start from a deep sleep, as though someone had shaken me. I sat up on my elbows, completely disoriented. I had a clear message in my head saying, *"You need to tell them how to get into the house!"*

I didn't know who "them" was, or why they would need that information, but it seemed important, so I did as instructed.

6:37 a.m. - Katy - text to person last texted (Tiffany):

> Ok code 2 key box in carport is [redacted]. I need help getting dressed. Wilcox [Hospital] because I'm super sick.

After that, I fell back into a semiconscious state.

The next text message on my phone to Tiffany is dated September 30th, two weeks later, thanking her for saving my life.

Tiffany to the Rescue

Tiffany lived 15 minutes away. After reading my texts, she rushed to my house as quickly as she could. She let herself in using the code I had just texted her. Without that code, she would have had no way to reach me in my upstairs bedroom in the house I had carefully locked up because I was home alone and feeling vulnerable.

Tiffany ran up the stairs, calling out as she came into my room. She found me barely responsive, sprawled on top of my covers.

The second memory I have of this morning was waking up to Tiffany crying out, "Oh my gosh, Katy, oh my gosh," over and over. She sounded desperate and terrified.

I remember trying to open my eyes and thinking to myself, "Wow. I must really be sick. She's freaking out!"

She struggled to help me sit up and tried to get me to stand. I don't remember any of this, but I do know from Tiffany that I was trying to stand on a broken foot, with no memory of having broken it.

"My feet hurt," I cried. "I can't stand up!"

"Why, what's wrong with your feet? What happened?"

"I think I fell," I sobbed.

These vague responses, slurred as if I were drunk, were out of character for me. Tiffany knew that I didn't drink alcohol and was cautious about medications, so this amplified her fear. But rather than press me for answers in my confused state, she shifted into problem-solving mode.

Grabbing a fuzzy blanket off the top of my bed, she wrapped it around me. Then she had me sit on the floor, and helped me scoot to the wooden stairway that leads from my bedroom to the main living area. She coached me to use my heels and pull myself across the wood floor, down my bedroom stairs, and down the second flight of stairs that leads to ground level. She helped me into the backseat of her truck, where she had blankets and pillows waiting to keep me warm on the one-hour drive to the hospital. I immediately lay down on the pillows and tried to rest.

Spooked by my condition, Tiffany wanted to call an ambulance. In my delirium, I objected that ambulances are expensive and it would wake and worry the whole neighborhood. I was still under the mistaken assumption that whatever I had was easily treatable, and I knew from experience that sirens echoed across the entire valley, alerting the whole community that someone was in trouble. I hated the thought of a neighbor calling Scott and worrying him unnecessarily.

Ignoring my objection, she called a firefighter friend to ask if he thought it was safe for her to take me to the hospital herself. He confirmed her suspicion that an ambulance would be at least 20 minutes away. If we waited for them at my house, we would be losing precious time getting to the hospital. He suggested driving toward Lihue and calling an ambulance along the way if I showed signs of distress. He reminded her to pay attention to mile markers in case she needed to call for help. At this point, I seemed to be alert and breathing normally, so Tiffany took off, checking in on me regularly to make sure my condition hadn't worsened.

On the drive to the hospital, Tiffany tried to reach Scott, but couldn't. He was still fishing on a remote river with no cell phone coverage. She knew my family well and suggested she call my 22-year-old daughter, Dani. I asked her to wait to call Dani until we knew what was happening. I didn't want to scare Dani or her 20-year-old sister, Jordan. Again, I recalled the trauma of Dani's friend going into septic shock and having one of her legs amputated below the knee. I didn't want to trigger that trauma for my girls when I was surely just in need of some extra fluids and bed rest.

I'm on Fire

About 15 minutes out from the hospital, everything changed.

I cried out in pain from the backseat, saying, "My hands and feet are on fire!" I begged her to go faster.

Tiffany knew it was time to reach out for help. She called ahead to the hospital and asked if they could meet us with a gurney at the ER entrance. After getting me in the car by herself, she knew she would need help getting me into the hospital, and my condition seemed to be worsening by the minute.

We couldn't imagine what was happening to my hands and feet that would be causing me so much pain. Tiffany realized this was not normal and that I needed medical help urgently. She drove as fast as she could safely drive.

As promised, medical staff met us at the emergency room entrance with a gurney. They rushed me into a room in the emergency department while Tiffany checked me in.

Wilcox Medical Center, Kauai

When we arrived at the hospital, Tiffany was able to convince the doctors that although I seemed "pleasant and talkative" (a quote from my medical chart), I had been wailing in the car just moments before. She recognized my typical minimizing behavior: feeling bad for causing these nice medical professionals all this trouble, I was trying to downplay my illness to relieve their distress. She made sure they understood that I was feeling *far* worse than I was admitting.

If Tiffany hadn't stayed with me, I would have wasted critical time in the waiting room because I wasn't acting as sick as I was. Valuable minutes that, as it turns out, were needed to save my life. She knew me well, and these doctors had just met me.

Per my medical chart, I was admitted to the emergency department at Wilcox Medical Center at 8:11 a.m. They took my vital signs and determined my breathing rate and heart rate were higher than normal. My temperature of 99° was slightly elevated, but it was still within normal range. My blood pressure, on the other hand, was 50/30 – so low I was immediately transferred from the emergency department to the ICU.

I didn't know it at the time, but I've since learned that a blood pressure that low is incompatible with life. My blood pressure is typically 120/86, so 50/30 was *way* too low for me. No wonder I wasn't thinking clearly, would pass out when I tried to stand, and felt like my hands were on fire! My body was sending signals that something had gone terribly wrong.

My suspected diagnosis was *sepsis*, the same condition that nearly cost Dani's friend her life. Per Sepsis Alliance (www.sepsis.org), "Sepsis is a life-threatening emergency that happens when your body's response to an infection damages vital organs and, often, causes death. In other words, it's your body's overactive and toxic response to an infection. Like strokes or heart attacks, sepsis is a medical emergency that requires rapid diagnosis and treatment." The diagnosis would need to be confirmed with blood work, which could take several hours. Time I didn't have.

Fortunately, Wilcox Medical Center had a well-rehearsed sepsis protocol.[1] As soon as my medical team suspected I might have sepsis, they sent my blood to the lab to check for specific indicators and identify if there was bacteria in my blood that was making me sick. I was given oxygen through a cannula, a plastic tube placed beneath my nostrils, to increase my low blood-oxygen levels. Large amounts of fluids were pumped into my body through an IV, and a flexible tube was placed in my vein to administer fluids and medications, in an attempt to increase my critically low blood pressure. I was also given the strongest available broad-spectrum antibiotics through the IV.

These IV antibiotics were potent and would be effective against many of the possible types of bacteria that may have triggered my illness, even MRSA (Methicillin-resistant Staphylococcus Aureus), which is resistant to many antibiotics, including the one I had been prescribed and began taking at home. If they could determine another cause of my low blood pressure, the antibiotics could be easily stopped or changed.

Administering fluids, oxygen, and antibiotics when sepsis is suspected is no guarantee, but it helps save lives. It can take hours to get bloodwork back from the lab, and days to identify a specific pathogen. My doctors knew that for every hour a patient with septic shock waits for an antibiotic, their chance of death increases significantly. If I were in septic shock, as they suspected, my organs were likely failing. Any delay in treatment could cost me my life.

Studies show that with sepsis, every hour a person waits to get treatment increases their chance of dying by 7.6%.[2] In my case, there was

---

1. https://www.sepsis.org/sepsis-basics/treatment/
2. Kumar, Anand MD; Roberts, Daniel MD; Wood, Kenneth E. DO; Light, Bruce

a possibility I'd had sepsis as early as the day before, meaning I'd already waited 10-15 hours before getting medical help. I was fighting for my life, and the odds were not in my favor.

When the bloodwork came back, it confirmed that I had several indicators consistent with sepsis. When this information was considered along with my vital signs and symptoms, I was diagnosed with the highest stage of sepsis: *septic shock.*

DIC - Death Is Coming

The pain in my hands and feet continued to worsen, suggesting a worrisome complication called Disseminated Intravascular Coagulation (DIC). DIC is so severe that the acronym has taken on an alternate meaning, "Death Is Coming." It causes bleeding and clotting within the capillaries in limbs and organs, disrupting vital blood flow. It can cause irreversible damage, including organ failure, amputations, and even death.

Even with advances in the diagnostics and treatment of sepsis, death rates associated with septic shock are as high as 30% to 50%.[3] According to the National Institute of Health, when sepsis is complicated by a diagnosis of DIC, the mortality rate doubles.[4] That means I had a 60% to 100% chance of dying.

Thankfully, I had no understanding of this at the time. My friends

---

MD; Parrillo, Joseph E. MD; Sharma, Satendra MD; Suppes, Robert BSc; Feinstein, Daniel MD; Zanotti, Sergio MD; Taiberg, Leo MD; Gurka, David MD; Kumar, Aseem PhD; Cheang, Mary MSc. Duration of hypotension before initiation of effective antimicrobial therapy is the critical determinant of survival in human septic shock. Critical Care Medicine 34(6):p 1589-1596, June 2006. | DOI: 10.1097/01.CCM.0000217961.75225.E9

3. Mahapatra S, Heffner AC. Septic Shock. [Updated 2023 Jun 12]. In: StatPearls [Internet]. Treasure Island (FL): StatPearls Publishing; 2025 Jan-. Available from: https://www.ncbi.nlm.nih.gov/books/NBK430939/

4. Unar A, Bertolino L, Patauner F, Gallo R, Durante-Mangoni E. Pathophysiology of Disseminated Intravascular Coagulation in Sepsis: A Clinically Focused Overview. Cells. 2023 Aug 22;12(17):2120. doi: 10.3390/cells12172120. PMID: 37681852; PMCID: PMC10486945.

who came to the hospital have told me I was blissfully unaware of the gravity of the situation. This was likely due to a combination of the inflammation in my body clouding my brain and the narcotic painkillers that were being administered for the pain in my hands and feet. Whatever the reason, I'm grateful.

My vital signs were monitored closely. As the day progressed, my blood-oxygen levels were decreasing, a sign that my lungs were failing. The cannula in my nostrils was replaced with a large mask that helped push oxygen into my lungs in hopes that the oxygen levels in my blood would increase.

My medical team was working with infectious disease specialists, trying to determine the exact strain of bacteria making me sick so they could target an antibiotic more likely to kill it. At the same time, they were considering the possibility that a fungus, parasite, or even a virus could be the source of the infection that caused me to go into septic shock.

Despite the efforts of some of the top infectious disease specialists in the state, we were never able to track down the exact pathogen that had triggered sepsis in my body. As it turns out, tracking down a specific pathogen is much more challenging than you might think. I had always imagined doctors put blood in a culture dish and it grows one or two clear pathogens, like the controlled experiments I did in high school chemistry. This is not the case. In as many as 50% of sepsis cases, doctors never find a clear cause.[5] For this reason, many patients must endure broad-spectrum antibiotics, which are less effective and trigger more side effects than a single targeted antibiotic.

Given the gaps in my memory, I've pieced together much of my journey through photos, videos, stories from friends who were there, and text messages on my phone and on the phones of my friends and family. When I look back at the photos I took that day, I can tell I was

5. Vincent JL. The Clinical Challenge of Sepsis Identification and Monitoring. PLoS Med. 2016 May 17;13(5):e1002022. doi: 10.1371/journal.pmed.1002022. PMID: 27187803; PMCID: PMC4871479.

taking pictures to share with my kids and husband, showing them how seriously the hospital was taking my condition. At the same time, I was trying to reassure them with my ubiquitous bright smile that I was going to be okay.

In reality, it was a miracle that I got to the hospital at all that morning. This story nearly ended before it began.

My gut instinct on Friday night was right. I *was* in grave danger, only the threat wasn't lurking in the shadows of my backyard. It was lurking inside my own body. And somehow, in the wee hours of Saturday morning, I intuitively understood that my only chance of survival was to reach out for help and get the medical care I was receiving from the doctors and nurses at Wilcox.

CHAPTER 5

THINGS ARE GETTING REAL

"Sometimes the strength within you is not a big, fiery flame for all to see; it is just a tiny spark that whispers ever so softly, You got this. Keep going!"

– Unknown

Sunday Afternoon, September 16, 2018

Tiffany & Friends

On that first day at Wilcox Medical Center on Kauai, Tiffany stayed by my side to act as my advocate and liaison to my family. Later that day, two other friends joined her. I wasn't thinking clearly and couldn't advocate effectively for myself, so I was fortunate to have my Kauai friends nearby to comfort me and ensure my unique needs were being met.

Dani - My Eldest Daughter

As soon as Tiffany heard my suspected diagnosis, she reached out to my eldest daughter, Dani, in San Diego. Dani was with her roommate when Tiffany called her from my phone. She picked up cheerfully, expecting to hear my voice. Instead, she heard Tiffany explain that I was in the hospital with possible septic shock.

Dani couldn't believe what she was hearing as Tiffany filled her in on what had happened and assured her that she and some of my other friends would remain with me until Scott or another family member could be by my side. Dani had been with me just a few days earlier, and now I might be in septic shock, of all things? She hadn't even heard of sepsis until three years prior, and now two of the closest people in the world to her had become critically ill from it. She prayed that my blood work would come back negative for sepsis and that this would all turn out to be a misunderstanding.

Tiffany emphasized that the doctors were concerned about my condition and they wanted to speak to Scott as soon as possible, so Dani immediately began trying to track down her father. She worried he would be difficult to reach because of the limited cell phone reception in the remote Idaho rivers where he was fishing. When her call went to voicemail, she hung up and sent him a text asking him to call her as soon as he received the message.

Unable to reach her dad, and knowing she would have to be stoic to get through the day, Dani set her emotions aside and shifted her focus to connecting with family and friends in his absence. As she made her list of people to contact, she realized several of them had a surprising amount of applicable knowledge and expertise. Aside from Marnie, mother of Julia (her friend who had survived sepsis), there was her aunt Maren, a former ER doctor, as well as Midori, my best friend and former neighbor, who had supported her cousin through sepsis 18 months earlier.

Holly - My Sister-in-Law

Dani's first call was to her Aunt Holly in Utah, whom she knew could help her reach Scott, since Holly knew the outfitter organizing his fishing trip. She assured Dani she would get a message to Scott as soon as possible, freeing Dani up to focus on informing other family members.

Jordan - My Youngest Daughter

Dani took a deep breath and called her sister Jordan, who at the time was a sophomore in college in Los Angeles.

"Mom's in the hospital," she announced in the calmest tone she could muster.

"What?? How is that possible? We saw her three days ago! She was fine."

Dani explained how I had called Tiffany, feeling like I had the flu and might be severely dehydrated. She hesitated to reveal more. She hated to scare her sister before she had additional information to pass on, but she knew Jordan would want the whole story.

Reluctantly, Dani went on, "The doctors think she may have septic shock, like Julia had."

The silence on the other end of the phone was deafening.

"Can you remember anything from that visit? Any symptoms Mom had while she was in L.A.? We need to give the doctors any information that might be useful."

"She seemed a little more tired than usual, I guess," Jordan replied. "I invited her to meet me for dinner on her last night in L.A., but she decided to just hang out in her hotel room instead. Which I thought was a little weird since she came all the way to California to see us. But, I mean, we'd spent a lot of time together over the past week, so I figured she just needed a vacation from her vacation."

Dani took notes to pass along to my medical care team and promised to let Jordan know of any changes in my condition.

Maren - My Sister-in-Law

Dani was anxious to talk to her Aunt Maren, who was a doctor trained in emergency medicine and was currently practicing clinical ethics and making documentary films at Stanford University. She knew she could help navigate the medical system and give an honest assessment of my health.

Dani was right. Maren immediately became a resource for medical advice and an advocate for our family. Her expertise was invaluable in helping our family navigate my health crisis.

Midori - Best Friend & Former Neighbor

It was a sunny Sunday in Seattle when Dani's name and photo popped up on Midori's phone. She answered excitedly, expecting an update on Dani's new job. She was wholly unprepared to hear Dani's shaky voice stating that I was in the ER on Kauai.

Confused by Dani's straightforward delivery, Midori confirmed, "She's in the emergency department?"

"Yes, she's in critical condition. They think it's septic shock."

Like my daughters, Midori had a hard time wrapping her mind around this sudden shift in my health status, and was stunned to hear Dani use the word "septic." She knew Julia had lost a leg to sepsis in college, and her cousin Lynn, who was like a sister to her, had nearly died from it just 18 months earlier. She couldn't believe this was happening again.

Midori recalled with trauma-induced clarity the day 18 months earlier when she'd received a similar phone call from her cousin's terrified husband. "Lynn has sepsis," he'd said. "She's on a business trip in North Carolina. She's unconscious in the ICU. They say she may not survive."

Midori had reached out to me on her way to North Carolina when Lynn was sick. I'd told her all I knew about Julia's narrow survival and ongoing fallout from sepsis, and recommended she talk with Julia's mom, Marnie. Marnie was an invaluable resource in helping Midori guide her family through Lynn's harrowing experience.

"Is she conscious?" she asked Dani.

"She is, but she's on oxygen, and her blood pressure is dangerously low." Dani went on to explain that Tiffany was with me but would need to leave in the evening, and she still couldn't reach Scott. Midori realized that, like her cousin Lynn, who ultimately lost her thumb in the ordeal and suffered nerve damage to her hand, I was going through the hell that is sepsis without family by my side. She knew right away what she had to do.

Because Midori had visited Kauai often, she was aware of the daily direct afternoon flight from Seattle to Kauai, which she might be able to catch if she hurried. Despite having less than two hours to get to the airport, she volunteered to fly to Hawaii to be with me and act as my advocate and family liaison until Scott could be by my side.

She wanted Dani and Jordan to know that I wouldn't be alone and that they would continue to receive regular updates on my condition. She also wanted to be sure I was receiving the best possible medical treatment. After her experience supporting Lynn, she understood the kind of help I would need.

She threw some clothes into a bag, grabbed her computer, and rushed to the airport. She would be on Kauai that evening to relieve Tiffany and my other friends so they could get some much-needed rest.

Knowing that Midori would be in Hawaii allowed Dani and Jordan to remain in California for work and school. Dani was starting a new job the next day, and Jordan's semester had just begun. They were hopeful and prayed that my condition would improve.

Marnie - Family Friend and Mother of Sepsis Survivor Julia

When Julia went into septic shock three years earlier, her mother, Marnie, stayed by her side in the ICU and throughout her entire recovery. During this time, Marnie became an expert on septic shock, ICUs, and many of the possible complications. Dani reached out to her as soon as she could for advice on what could be done for sepsis and how to navigate the medical system during recovery.

Marnie was heartbroken that this was happening to me and volunteered to do everything she could, including offering to fly to Hawaii if help was needed while I was in the hospital. She comforted Dani, hoping my situation would be less critical and more treatable than Julia's. Marnie was anxious to talk to Scott, Midori, and Maren to share her invaluable advice.

When Marnie passed the news on to Julia, her first response was disbelief. The doctors had impressed upon her that sepsis was less likely in a healthy person who was neither very old nor very young,[1] yet it had happened to her. Now here it was happening again, to me of all people. She'd known me since she and Dani had become fast friends on the first day of kindergarten and she thought of me as a second mother. She knew how committed I was to my health and had seen me just a few months prior on another mainland visit, looking happy and fit. What were the odds?

She told herself it must be a mistake, that they would get more information soon and discover it wasn't sepsis after all. Because if it was, she knew better than anyone what a long, hard road might lie ahead for all of us.

Scott - My Husband

Scott had been looking forward to an extended fishing trip on the mainland. Hawaii is beautiful and has a lot of outdoor activities, but trout fishing isn't one of them. He planned to fish with his brothers in Idaho for a long weekend, then take off on a road trip to several fly-fishing rivers in Montana and Wyoming.

---

1. Adults over 65 are 13 times more likely to be hospitalized with sepsis than adults under 65 (https://www.cdc.gov/nchs/products/databriefs/db62.htm), but more than 42,000 children, most under the age of 5, also develop severe sepsis each year and 4,400 of them die, more than from cancer (https://academic.oup.com/bjaed/article-abstract/4/1/12/356894?redirectedFrom=fulltext).

This trip was to be a solo adventure to work on his fly-fishing skills and contemplate the next phase of his life as he headed into retirement and Empty Nest territory. Like me, he was searching for direction, and this fishing trip was his version of my Greek Goddess odyssey.

He was just winding down his first day of fishing with his young guide when they floated into cell range, and the guide's phone pinged with a message.

Scott was startled when the guide turned to him and asked, "Is your wife Katy?"

"Yes, why?" The guide handed the phone to Scott so he could read the text that had just arrived from our sister-in-law Holly, explaining that I was currently in the ICU on Kauai with probable septic shock, and he should call her or Dani immediately.

He saw the words but couldn't comprehend how this was possible, given that he had just spoken with me two days earlier and had received a text from me the previous night. I had told him about the blister on my finger, but said I would start taking oral antibiotics over the weekend if it got worse. My text from the night before said I was too tired to talk and that I would talk to him the next day, but gave no indication that I was getting sick, let alone critically ill. He couldn't fathom how I could now be in the ICU, only 12 hours after he had last heard from me.

Reflexively, Scott latched on to the positive aspects of what he'd heard. Yes, it sounded serious, but I was in the ICU, the best place to handle a medical emergency. I had friends with me. He told himself everything was going to be okay.

Still, he was deeply shaken by the news and said to the guide, "I'm sorry to do this, but we've got to push out." After a long, hard row back to the takeout point ashore, Scott phoned Dani and told her he would get to Hawaii as soon as he could. He was relieved when Dani told him that Midori was already on a flight to Hawaii and would be with me that evening, and that Maren was checking in with Tiffany regularly to help manage my care.

After filling him in on my condition, Dani said she and Jordan were ready to go to Hawaii if he thought it was a good idea. He asked her to wait until he could see me for himself. Like the girls, he was hoping my condition would improve by the time he got there. On the off-chance it didn't, he didn't want the girls to be there without him.

He tried calling the hospital to reach me directly, but couldn't. He tried calling Tiffany, but she was so busy keeping friends and family informed about the situation that it took several tries before he could reach her. When he finally did, he told her he was on his way and would arrive the next morning. She was relieved to know that he had finally been reached and promised she would stay with me until Midori arrived. She updated him on my status and said there was talk of trying to get me to The Queen's Medical Center on Oahu if my condition continued to deteriorate.

He asked her to pass the phone to me, then to go and bring my doctor into the room so he could talk to him. I remember this phone call because it confused and scared me. I had been waiting all day to talk to Scott and was excited that he was finally calling, but he was so serious on the phone, and I didn't understand why. I wasn't thinking clearly, and had no idea how dire and stressful the situation was.

"How are you feeling?" Scott asked in a grave tone.

I told him the pain in my hands and feet was excruciating, but that the medicine they were giving me in my IV was making it bearable.

"Stay strong. I love you, and I'll be with you as soon as I possibly can." His voice was very strained.

When the doctor arrived in the room, Scott directed me to tell him that Dr. Maren Monsen, my sister-in-law, had my permission to make medical decisions for me and speak on my behalf.

I told him I would do it, and he said very sternly, "Katy, look at him now, while I'm on the phone, and say, 'I give my permission for my sister-in-law, Dr. Maren Monsen, to be my medical advisor to speak on my behalf.' "

I did as he said, and the doctor acknowledged that he'd be happy to speak with Maren regarding my medical care. This conversation was noted in my chart.

Had he not insisted I say those words right away, with him as a witness, there's a good chance I would have forgotten what to say or to say anything at all.

Hawaii Bound

Scott and his brothers packed up immediately and began the long drive back to Salt Lake City, where Dani had booked him on the earliest available flight to Hawaii, departing the next morning.

Scott's brother drove the rental car so Scott could coordinate with our daughters and my doctors whenever they were in cell range. He was frustrated and felt helpless because of the poor cell coverage while driving over mountain passes and through remote areas during the six-hour drive.

When he finally came to a spot with decent service, Scott asked his brother to pull over. He started making phone calls right there, on the side of the interstate. He finally reached Maren, who updated him on my condition.

"They're doing everything I would do," she reassured him, but emphasized that it was dire. "I'm glad you'll be with her as soon as you can get there. Tell the girls to come as soon as they can too."

He also had text messages on his phone from Marnie offering her sepsis and patient advocacy expertise. He reached out to her by text, and she gave him great advice, including questions to ask my doctors, and helpful things to do for me while I was in the hospital. She assured him she was on-call and available 24 hours a day to help however she could.

A Matter of Life and Death

Though I knew I was being given antibiotics for an infection and that coming to the hospital was the right call, I had no true understanding of my situation. My medical charts and the information I got from friends and family would later enlighten me about the gravity of my condition in those first 24 hours of treatment. Throughout that day, many of my organs began to fail from poor blood flow, inflammation, and lack of oxygen, including my kidneys, liver, lungs, and even my heart.

By the end of my first day in the hospital, I was diagnosed with several serious complications of septic shock: MODS (Multi-Organ Dysfunction Syndrome), SIRS (Systemic Inflammatory Response Syndrome), and ARDS (Acute Respiratory Distress Syndrome).[2] My blood pressure remained unstable throughout the day despite the IV fluid being administered. My failing kidneys were unable to process the fluid, causing my body to swell significantly. I eventually gained 30 pounds from fluid retention, almost as much weight as I gained during each of my full-term pregnancies.

It was becoming increasingly clear that I needed to be transferred to a larger hospital on Oahu, better equipped to handle the severity of my illness. My friends and family had been researching hospitals in Hawaii. They wanted me to be transferred to The Queen's Medical Center in Honolulu because it was a level-one trauma center with an impeccable reputation. Additionally, Queen's had hyperbaric chambers[3] readily available that could help my hands and feet, as well as my vital organs, to recover from the severe damage they'd sustained in my sepsis battle.

When my medical team called for a transfer, though, there were no

2. A condition similar to SARS (Severe Acute Respiratory Syndrome), caused by the coronavirus, COVID-19.

3. Hyperbaric chambers are pressurized oxygen chambers commonly used to help scuba divers who have ascended too quickly and developed "the bends."

open beds in the ICU at Queen's. We would have to hope my condition remained stable long enough for a bed to become available.

Midori

Midori arrived from Seattle on Sunday night, allowing my Kauai friends to return home and to their families. She stayed by my bed, comforting me throughout the night.

At my request, she held my hands and feet to warm them because I felt like they were frozen. She could see they were beginning to turn purple at my wrists, and that the bruise-like discoloration was slowly growing toward my palms.

"Remember that snowboarding trip when the weather was so horrible and I got frostbite on my toes? It feels like that, only worse," she later recalled me telling her.

I don't remember the pain that night in the hospital, but I will never forget the snowboarding trip when the temperature was -30° with wind chill, and it felt like knives stabbing my toes as they warmed up. If I was experiencing that excruciating pain again, and it wasn't going away as it had after snowboarding, no wonder they couldn't block it with even the most potent painkillers.

To try to distract me and help pass the time, Midori read me articles about health, fitness, and nutrition, my recent passions. It broke her heart to see me in such dire straits. I was so much sicker than she had imagined. Just as she had with her cousin Lynn, she watched my vitals on the monitors with more anxious attention than a team owner watching a tight score at the Super Bowl. She wanted me transferred to a larger hospital as soon as possible, but "best friend and neighbor" didn't have legal standing to advocate on my behalf.

I can't remember her being there at all. These memory gaps frustrate me, and I briefly considered doing hypnotherapy to try to recapture those missing memories. Still, Midori and my family have assured me it's for the best that I can't remember that scary time and the agonizing pain. I know they're right, and now I see my lack of recollection of that difficult time as a blessing.

I have a photo of Midori on my phone: she's sitting next to my hospital bed, texting with my family. I'm sure she was overwhelmed, trying to be present and keep me comfortable while also communicating with my entire family, all of whom felt anxious, concerned, and helpless not to be by my side. I'm so appreciative that she was there with me when my family couldn't be.

Scott

When he got cell service near Salt Lake City, Scott called Midori. That's when he heard about the discoloration on my hands and feet.

Throughout the day, I had been taking pictures on my phone showing my hands and feet slowly turning purple, with little patchy bruises and thick red lines at the center of my wrist extending toward my palm. This was an indicator of permanent tissue damage, but I was still unaware that something so serious was happening to me. I just thought of it as bruising that would surely heal as normal bruises do.

With this news, Scott was concerned that my hands and feet were in dire straits, like Julia's foot had been. The pressure was mounting for me to get to Oahu.

My family and friends prayed for my body to become strong enough to be transported. Meanwhile, Maren tapped into her network of medical professionals, reaching out to a colleague who had direct connections with the ICU head at The Queen's Medical Center. She emphasized the urgency of my situation and our desire to be at Queen's. She pushed to see if they could find space for me in the ICU, knowing that less critical patients could sometimes be moved out of the ICU to make room for sicker patients.

Dani remained the main point of contact for other family members to find out how I was doing. She kept Jordan closely in the loop and promised to let her know when she had more information. She was hoping Jordan could stay focused on school as the semester had just begun, and junior year was notoriously challenging.

They were both in a holding pattern, praying that my condition would turn around and they could put this scare behind them. At the ages of 20 and 22, they had been forced to step up and become my guardians while they couldn't reach their father.

This was the day my girls truly became adults.

When Scott reached out to the hospital, he was notified that my condition was progressively worsening. My medical team was concerned about fluid retention because my kidneys were no longer functioning, and my lungs, hands, and feet were suffering severe damage. My extremities had turned magenta overnight with grotesque red blotches moving from my fingers and toes into my hands and feet. This was an indication that my circulation was being affected by the DIC, along with the vasopressors[4] used to move blood from my extremities into my vital organs (brain, heart, kidneys, and lungs) to keep me alive. We hadn't confirmed it at the time, but there were indications that my liver and digestive system might also be impacted.

Getting me to Honolulu as soon as possible had become a matter of life and death.

---

4. Patients are placed on vasopressors when their blood pressure is so dangerously low that their vital organs are not receiving enough oxygen rich blood and therefore cannot function. The blood is then shunted away from the hands and feet to the vital organs. If the blood pressure to vital organs is not improved it can cause permanent organ damage such as brain damage, kidney failure or even heart failure.

CHAPTER 6

TRUSTING THE PROCESS

"Whenever the rainbow appears in the clouds, I will see it. I remember the everlasting covenant between God and all living creatures of every kind on the Earth."

– The Holy Bible, Genesis 9:11–16

Monday Morning, September 17, 2018

4:45 a.m. - Valorie (friend) - text to Katy:

> Sweetie, I'll be in about 12-ish today. How is your pain in your stomach

4:49 am - from Katy

> The stomach is better. Now it's feet and dis I fort [discomfort] with lungs. You are so sweet. Only come if you are near here. Talking strains my oxygen levels. But I would love to see you. 💕

4:50 am - from Valorie

OK praying for U my friend 🩶🩶🩶

The pain in my stomach caused my doctors a lot of searching and testing as they tried to eliminate something internal that may have been the real source of my infection. The wound on my thumb was relatively small, so they feared it may have been a secondary source of infection, with the primary source being a more serious infection within my body.

They ruled out the possibility of a urinary tract infection and anything involving my reproductive system. They also confirmed I had not forgotten to remove a tampon that could have caused toxic shock syndrome.[1]

They did scans of my body to determine if there was an infection in my lungs, liver, kidneys, stomach, or heart, but found nothing. They also ruled out any chance of an infection in my mouth that might have come from a recently pulled tooth and bone graft.

Since they still couldn't tell what type of bacteria was making me sick, they would need to continue treating me with the most potent antibiotics, which would take a greater toll on my body.

Scott

Scott flew from Salt Lake City to Los Angeles, then boarded a flight to Honolulu. Before losing cell coverage over the Pacific Ocean, he made a few quick phone calls, managing logistics with Midori, Maren, Holly, and our girls.

1. Toxic shock syndrome, or TSS, became well known in the early 1980s after the development of a highly absorbent tampon designed to prevent leakage, allowing women the convenience of going a full day without changing the tampon. Unfortunately, it was so absorbent that women were leaving tampons in their bodies longer than recommended, causing bacterial infections that triggered a surge in cases of toxic shock syndrome. The symptoms of toxic shock and septic shock are slightly different, but close enough that I could have had either.

Scott - text to Katy (through Midori):

> I just got wi-fi so I'm aware of what's happening. I love you so much. I'm talking to our girls. They are coming over to see you, flying in tonight. They are amazing. You should be very proud of how they are handling all of this.

> You're an amazing wife and incredible mother. Now it's time to be selfish. Just focus on your recovery. Nothing else. Tell your body to get better. Love you. Love you. 😍😍🩶🩶

Scott - text to Dani and Jordan:

> I'm so thankful you both are coming. I texted your mom and told her you both will be by her side in a few hours. It meant the world to her. I know this trip is difficult. It significantly impacts your lives and it will be difficult seeing your mom in an ICU. I am so thankful for and inspired by your courage and selflessness: reminds me so much of who your mom is. None of us would be who we are without her. It's time for us three to give back a small part of the endless sacrifice she made for us. Thanks for actively being a part of that. Love you guys.

Scott was grateful he had been bumped up to first class, so he only had one other person sitting next to him on the flight. When he hung up his phone and set it in his lap, the man next to him said, "Excuse me, I couldn't help but overhear that your wife is in critical condition. I'm so sorry for all that you're going through. I wanted to tell you that I've been where you are right now."

Before Scott could react, the man explained that several years earlier, his young son had been in a motorcycle accident in the U.K. He had to fly to him on a plane that also had no Wi-Fi, then he sat helplessly by his son's side in the ICU for many weeks, hearing again and again that his son was unlikely to survive. He and his family prayed and held out hope that he would recover.

He said he just wanted Scott to know that his son eventually awoke from his coma, and that after spending time in physical therapy and allowing his brain to heal, his son had recovered fully and was leading a happy and productive life.

"I'm sorry for intruding," he told Scott, "but I just wanted you to know that miracles do happen."

Scott was touched that he had shared this personal story. They continued to talk about their lives, allowing Sott to relax after the frustration of realizing he would have several hours without status updates. He was grateful for the hope this stranger offered that even in my grave condition, I could still recover.

Midori

After a restless night at the hospital on Kauai, Midori finally received word that a room was available in the ICU at The Queen's Medical Center, and I would be transported later that morning. This was the answer to our collective prayers.

Many things needed to be coordinated for my transfer, which took several hours. Midori could see everyone bustling around me, doing tests and changing out the various machines connected to me with tubing and electrical lines. She heard talk of coordinating the ambulance from the hospital to make connections with the air ambulance, scheduled for later that morning. If all went well, we would arrive in Honolulu around the same time as Scott's connecting flight from Los Angeles.

Midori was relieved that Scott would be meeting us at Queen's. Having Scott there meant more than just having my husband with me, it meant having someone present with the authority to make medical decisions on my behalf.

Katy

I have very few memories of this time, but I do remember my doctor explaining to me on Monday morning that it would be safest for me to have a breathing tube inserted in my mouth so a machine could breathe for me while I was in transit. This intubation would require me to be placed in a coma to make the journey safer. The doctor said that they would give me medication to knock me out, put a tube down my throat into my trachea, and place me on a ventilator. He explained that this would help my oxygen levels and said that I would not feel a thing.

Knowing it would be a relief to no longer feel like I was struggling for air or enduring the constant aching pain in my hands and feet, I gratefully agreed.

I had no idea that might have been the last time I would ever be conscious again.

I have since learned that one of the most dangerous times for any patient is when they are transferred from one hospital to another. In my case, that concern was outweighed by the fact that if they didn't transfer me, I was likely to die.

Maren advised me over the phone to sign the paperwork. I did as she said. I know this because I've looked over my medical charts, and seen where I sloppily signed my name, giving consent to be intubated for the flight to Oahu.

Midori assured me she would not leave me until I was safely at Queen's in the care of their intensivists (ICU doctors), and Scott was by my side. I remember feeling happy that I would be flying to Oahu and thinking everything would be fine once I got there and could be with Scott.

Once intubated, I would be transferred by ambulance to the Kauai airport and then by a specially equipped airplane to the island of Oahu. Highly specialized flight paramedics would attend to me during the flight. I would then be loaded into a third ambulance that would drive me to the hospital we were counting on to save my life.

Scott

Scott occupied himself on the plane by writing long texts to the girls, thanking them for being so strong through this horrible experience. He also wrote texts to some of our close friends, letting them know what was happening. He knew any texts he wrote on the plane would be sent once he landed on Oahu.

As his flight finally approached Honolulu, Scott received a text from Midori informing him that I had been intubated and was being prepared for transport to The Queen's Medical Center. Based on the expected timing of my arrival, he would beat me there, giving him time to get situated and possibly check in with the ICU team before I arrived.

The Transfer

Midori was told she could accompany me in the tiny air ambulance, but would only be allowed to bring one bag, which she would need to carry in her lap. She had packed quickly in her haste to leave Seattle, using one suitcase for clothing and another suitcase for her computer and work-related items. She quickly shuffled the essentials into one of the bags and gave her extra suitcase to Tiffany, who promised she would bring it to her on Oahu or mail it wherever it needed to go.

An ambulance crew arrived to transport me to the airport as soon as my intubation was safely completed. I have since seen the video Midori took of my gurney being loaded into the ambulance near the emergency room at Wilcox Hospital. It's surreal for me to look back and see the red lights flashing as I'm being loaded into an ambulance, realizing I was the emergency inside.

When we arrived at the airport, Midori and I were transferred into the small air ambulance that would fly us to Oahu. The mood was tense in the airplane as Midori sat out of the way with her bag perched on her lap. They were having difficulty controlling my blood pressure and oxygen levels, and the eerie sound of the ventilator was a constant reminder that I wasn't breathing on my own.

In an attempt to distract Midori, one of the pilots suggested she look out the front window and take photos and videos, as this was a unique chance to see some of the shores of Kauai that commercial planes aren't allowed to fly over. She was grateful for the distraction of that stunning aerial view as they passed over the many beautiful beaches we had visited together in happier times.

Early in my recovery, when I was out of critical care, I asked my family to show me videos of the things I couldn't remember. That video of my intubated body inside a tiny airplane, my chest rising and falling with the mechanical rhythm of the ventilator, was both shocking and fascinating to me. I watched it over and over, realizing how extremely sick I had been. That undeniable physical evidence of my illness was invaluable when ICU delirium struck, and I couldn't recall why I was in the hospital.

When we landed at Honolulu International Airport, Midori and I were whisked into another ambulance. My gurney, IV, oxygen, and the equipment monitoring my vital signs were moved from the small airplane into the waiting ambulance. Midori noticed that the activity and tension in the ambulance were increasing as the lights and sirens were turned on and we raced into the city. She kept her fear at bay by taking another video from inside the ambulance.

In that video, I'm lying on the stretcher in the care of a paramedic with the sound of a siren in the background and red and blue lights reflecting off the highway signs as we raced to Honolulu. I had driven this road many times over the years when visiting Honolulu for my girls' soccer tournaments, holiday shopping trips, or big concerts. On every trip there, traffic had been bumper to bumper, as one would expect in any major metropolitan city. But not that day. I still get goosebumps and a lump in my throat when I remember seeing the video showing the cars in front of us peeling out of the way of our ambulance as we sped through the traffic, headed to Queen's. The urgency is palpable.

But then, as we emerge from the underpass, a vast, bright rainbow appears over Honolulu. No rain is visible, only an iridescent rainbow reaching from the lush green mountains in the center of the island to the tall buildings of downtown Honolulu and the hospital ahead.

Midori and I had first met almost 20 years earlier at a church we attended with our families near Seattle. We became friends in a women's Bible study, and we both knew that, in the Bible, a rainbow symbolizes grace, mercy, and hope. When she saw that rainbow over Honolulu, Midori took this as a sign that God had heard our prayers and everything would be okay. She held on to that sign as a promise from God that I would survive. She shared the story with Scott and our girls to remind them that we were not in this alone and that they should continue to hold out hope for my recovery.

CHAPTER 7

FOR BETTER OR FOR WORSE

"How queer everything is today! And yesterday, things went on just as usual. I wonder if I've been changed in the night?"

– Alice in Wonderland (Lewis Carroll, *Alice Through the Looking Glass*)

Monday, September 17 - The Queen's Medical Center, Oahu

When Scott arrived at Queen's, he went straight to the Intensive Care Unit, where a locked door confronted him.

"I'm here to see Katy Grainger. I'm her husband," he told the nurse who answered the door when he rang the buzzer at the entrance.

"She hasn't arrived yet," she told him, instructing him to sit in a chair just outside the ICU and wait for my arrival. There was no time for emotion as he continued texting friends and family, letting them know I was being transferred to Oahu and reassuring them that he would be by my side when I arrived. Based on Maren's recommendation, the girls were already on their way to Honolulu and would arrive later that night.

Within an hour, Scott received a text from Midori saying we had arrived at the hospital's ambulance bay. Moments later, an entourage of medical professionals rushed around the corner toward the ICU, escorting my gurney. Scott recognized the uniforms of EMTs, doctors, and nurses, all with serious expressions, like something out of a Hollywood medical drama. He was struck by how young they all seemed, like kids he could have coached just a few years ago. The scene was surreal. Then, as if to settle any question as to whether or not it was really his wife on that gurney, Midori appeared, following closely but careful to stay out of the way.

As I came into view on the gurney, Scott was stunned. I was barely recognizable. My face, neck, and body were swollen from the resuscitation fluids I'd been given that my damaged kidneys were unable to process. My eyes were taped shut, a breathing tube obscured my gaping mouth, and my chest rose and fell mechanically in sync with the whooshing sound of the ventilator that was breathing for me. He knew it was me, but had a hard time reconciling what he saw with the healthy, vital woman he had last seen on Kauai.

Scott rushed to my side but was stopped by an older doctor who asked, "Who are you?"

"I'm her husband," he replied desperately.

The doctor pointed to the chair where Scott had just been sitting and said, "Wait here. She's not stable."

He could barely hear the doctor saying something about updating him soon as he disappeared through the security doors of the intensive care unit.

Waiting for the Unknown

In a helpless daze, Scott sat down with Midori and texted Maren the update that I had arrived, but was "not stable." He couldn't bring himself to ask her what that might mean. Instead, he focused on the fact that all those medical professionals who had just rushed me into the ICU were doing everything they could to stabilize me. And when they succeeded, he would be there, ready and waiting.

Maren called him immediately and asked if they had confirmed that I had DIC. Scott didn't know for sure, but said he would ask when the doctor returned. He promised to keep her in the loop as he learned more. Maren reassured him that I was in the best place to get the care I needed.

While they anxiously awaited a status update from my doctor, Midori gave Scott the details of her time with me at Wilcox and our transport to Queen's. After about two hours, an unbearably long time, the doctor returned and reintroduced himself as my lead intensivist (critical care doctor).

"Your wife is very sick," he explained. "We are going to do all we can for her. In the meantime, if you have children or other people who would want to be here, you should call them and have them come immediately." He was about to return to the ICU when Scott remembered to ask Maren's question:

"Has it been confirmed that she has DIC?"

"Yes, she is in septic shock with DIC."

Scott didn't comprehend how serious the DIC diagnosis was until he relayed this information to Maren. He understood that it was impacting the circulation in my hands and feet. Still, he didn't realize that the same clotting and discoloration that was occurring in my hands and feet was impacting all of my internal organs with an equal ferocity, significantly decreasing my chances of survival.

Maren's response, "I'll leave for Honolulu as soon as I can," shocked Scott. He knew she had a busy week at work and hadn't planned to come over.

A shiver ran down his spine as he took in the urgency of her response and what that must mean for me. Suddenly aware that I was much sicker than he'd realized, Scott confronted the reality that he would now have to pass that dire news on to our girls.

Sitting outside the ICU with Midori, trying to process the fact that even Maren seemed to fear that I may not survive, Scott finally allowed the stress of the prior 24 hours to catch up to him and his emotions came flooding out in a torrent of tears. Midori comforted him, setting aside her emotions to focus on what needed to be done to prepare for the girls' arrival. After about 15 minutes, with a plan in place, she reminded him, "You need to get yourself together before the girls get here."

He knew she was right. He didn't have the luxury of falling apart. He would have to be strong for our daughters.

Midori told Scott she would give him some time alone at the hospital while she went to the hotel to check into the room that a friend had generously arranged for her and the girls. She encouraged him to stay at the hospital as long as he needed and assured him she would be there for Dani and Jordan when they arrived.

Alone with the gravity of the situation, Scott sent a difficult text to my parents and older brothers, who were anxiously awaiting word of my status.

> Hey Terry, it's been really rough here. There has been a downturn in her condition significant enough that they decided to airlift her to Queens med ctr on Oahu. She is now there and fully intubated. Several significant problems with her. It's very, very concerning. I'm here now. Dani and Jordan will be flying into Oahu tonight to join me and Midori so she has both advocacy and support. While her condition is extremely serious; this is exactly what ICUs specialize in treating, so she is in the right place. I will update you as I know more.

My parents were in their 80's and found it difficult to travel, but they had offered to come to Oahu if Scott thought they should. He asked them to wait so the girls could have some time alone with me, hoping my parents could visit when I was recovering. Had they been younger, they would have been on the first plane to Hawaii, but they knew I was in good hands with Scott and Maren overseeing my medical care and agreed to remain in Spokane until further notice.

In Sickness and In Health

Scott couldn't believe our lives had changed so drastically in 24 hours. Yesterday, he was fly-fishing in a tranquil Idaho river, and now he was 3,000 miles from there, alone in a strange hospital as the mother of his children was fighting for her life in the next room.

Our love story is, in many ways, a classic. We were high school sweethearts.

We met on the first day of my sophomore year of high school when Scott transferred to the small private school I had attended since 5th grade. My school bus was filled with younger kids, so I was thrilled when this handsome new guy stepped aboard. I later learned he was a junior who wouldn't turn 16 for a few more weeks, so he'd be riding my bus until he could get his license. Lucky me.

Scott was smart, witty, and approachable. We had math class together and several free periods throughout the week when we sat with each other in the upper school courtyard with classmates, laughing and joking while pretending to work on assignments.

At first, we were just friends. He had a girlfriend who still attended his former school, so there was no awkward pressure on our friendship. I could tell he was loyal to her, so it felt safe to spend time alone with him.

When he got his driver's license and offered me an alternative to taking the bus, it was an easy yes. Driving to and from school together every day, Scott became one of my closest friends.

When he and his girlfriend broke up near the end of the school year, our relationship remained platonic. That is, until I got strep throat and ended up missing a month of school. This was long before social media, cell phones, and texting, so I had no way of communicating with my friends. I missed all of them terribly, but most of all, I realized how much I missed Scott.

He brought me homework a couple of times a week, and we'd talk while he stood on my front porch. I was sad every time he left and couldn't wait to see him again.

When I finally returned to school, I knew my feelings for him had changed, and I was overjoyed when he asked me on our first date. By the time we went to prom together a month later, it was clear to everyone that we were not just an item, we were a committed couple.

We went to the University of Washington together, got engaged a year after graduating, and were married nine months later in Spokane, where our love had first blossomed. The lilacs were in full bloom, seven years and 20 days after our first date, as we vowed to love one another "in sickness and health, as long as we both shall live."

We have had a wonderful marriage, but it wasn't always easy. As we embarked on our career paths and became parents, we faced challenges that were far more difficult than the hiccups we'd overcome in college. While I was struggling through postpartum depression and confronting a recent diagnosis of ADHD, Scott was drowning in work stress and self-medicating with alcohol. The volatility of that combination nearly broke us.

That's when we realized it wasn't enough just to prioritize our partnership and family. We also needed to prioritize ourselves individually by getting the help we needed to heal and grow. We came out the other side stronger than ever – as people, as partners, and as parents.

We committed to strengthening ourselves individually so that we could be the pillars supporting our family. I hired a life coach to help me manage my chaotic days. She and I began with the basics like organizing my home office so I could easily pay bills, schedule chores, keep track of kids' activities, and plan shopping and nightly meals. Then I found ways to enrich my life through quality time with other parents, stroller walks with my best friend, and babysitting swaps with friends to make time to work out and go to appointments.

Scott stayed home in the mornings for an extra hour to help with breakfast and our morning routine, then shortened his days to be with the kids and help with dinner. When the girls were in elementary school, he began coaching soccer after school and continued until both girls graduated high school with state championships under their belts. As a family, we became more involved with our church, which provided community and spiritual enrichment for all of us.

Through small efforts and changes in each of our lives, we shifted the course of our marriage and family. After all we had overcome together as young parents, we felt like we could conquer anything. Anything, that is, but the one thing even our vows acknowledged could part us.

As Long as We Both Shall Live

After what seemed like hours, Scott was finally invited into the ICU to be by my side. With the nurses' permission, he gently held my discolored hands. He rested his forehead against mine and whispered that everything would be okay. Now that he was finally by my side, he allowed himself to cry again, quietly praying that his promise to me would be true.

The doctors and nurses came and went, updating Scott on any new information from the many tests they were performing. They reassured him that I was in the best place possible and that the top specialists available would be involved in my care. He felt comforted that so many capable medical professionals were doing all that they could to keep me alive.

When the intensivist returned after reviewing my lab work, Scott asked the doctor to give Maren the medical update he knew was coming.

"My sister-in-law is a doctor, so she'll understand what you're saying, and she can take her time explaining it to me so you can get back to work." The doctor agreed and spoke with Maren for about 10 minutes.

Before heading back into the ICU, he returned Scott's phone and asked, "Are your daughters on their way?"

"They are," Scott replied.

"Good," was the last word the doctor said before returning through the locked doors of the ICU.

As gently as possible, Maren explained to Scott that I was having difficulty keeping my blood pressure and oxygen levels in a safe range and that my kidneys and lungs were showing significant signs of failure.

"She's really, really sick, Scott."

"So what do we do? How do we get her better?" Scott was still in problem-solver mode and wanted instructions to follow. Instead, Maren confirmed his greatest fear.

"Scott… she might not make it."

Overwhelmed by the gravity of the situation, he tried to find other explanations for what he was hearing. His mind bounced between dozens of questions: Were *all* of my organs failing? Could I have brain damage because of a lack of oxygen, since my lungs weren't working well? How could this all happen so quickly? What were they doing to help my plum-colored hands? Could they stop my mottled feet from losing circulation like my hands? How was he going to tell the girls how sick I was?

And the worst thought of all: *Would I still be alive when the girls arrived?*

Maren asked if I had signed legal documents stating my wishes about receiving life support and designating a representative since I was unable to speak for myself. Scott couldn't believe what he was hearing. He went numb.

We had each signed Medical Directives when we had prepared our first Wills as young parents. We had conversations over the years about scenarios in which we would want to survive and the difficult scenarios where we would want the other person to withdraw life support and let us go. We were both clear that if either one of us suffered irreversible brain damage, we would not want to live. We both agreed that if the quality of either of our lives was so damaged that we would no longer be ourselves, neither of us would want to be kept on life support.

We had also signed Powers of Attorney, giving each other the right to make these decisions on our behalf if we were unable to do so ourselves. We were counting on each other to make that difficult choice, in line with our wishes. It terrified him that he might be asked to make this horrible decision for me since I was unable to speak for myself.

Joel - Close Family Friend

Scott stepped outside my room and called our dear friend Joel on Kauai. He asked if Joel could go to our home to retrieve my Will, Power of Attorney, and Medical Directive from our files. Joel was like a brother to us and would do anything for our family. He was anxious to help and said he would hop on a plane and deliver them personally.

Joel knew how serious septic shock could be. Five years earlier, his mother had been airlifted from Kauai in septic shock from an unknown infection. When we realized how sick Joel's mother was, Scott immediately booked a ticket and flew to Oahu to support Joel while he was waiting for his brothers to arrive from the mainland. It was mind-boggling that roles were now reversed, and Joel was doing the same for Scott and me.

Joel was grateful for an opportunity to let Scott know he wasn't alone. He was scared for my life but held out hope that if his mother could survive septic shock, so could I.

Dani and Jordan

Dani and Jordan had departed for Hawaii just before Scott had a chance to assess my condition. All they knew when their plane took off from Los Angeles was that I had been intubated and was on my way to a hospital on Oahu that was better equipped to care for me. They were comforted knowing Midori was by my side and Scott might be able to arrive at the hospital before me.

They learned during that long flight what it meant to let go of control and give a situation over to God. They prayed nonstop that by the time they arrived, my condition would have improved. They held out hope that I would be fine.

Although they had flown back and forth between Hawaii and the mainland many times over the years, that flight felt torturously long.

When they landed, the girls saw a text from Scott.

> I am very proud of you both… your initiative and take-charge approach yesterday, while I was unavailable, was incredible. Your level-headedness in evaluating your priorities is smart and appropriate. You are both handling this crisis very well. With initiative and clarity. Thank you.

> The doctors are still getting Mom situated in the ICU after her flight. There is an enormous amount of things that need to be done with machine hookups, monitors, medication, etc. They need to finish that tonight and then the doctors are requiring uninterrupted rest. So we will come to the hospital to see her tomorrow.

He followed up with a text saying Midori was at the hotel and that he would meet them there so I could rest for the night.

Chan - Dani's friend from Kauai

Chan, who was attending the University of Hawaii, met the girls at the airport and took them to The Royal Hawaiian Hotel on Waikiki Beach. They had walked through the beautiful grounds of the hotel before, but had never stayed there. They felt comforted by the tropical park-like setting and iconic pink stucco buildings. They knew our close friend had arranged it for them as a place to relax after traveling home under such difficult circumstances, which made it feel even more special.

Midori greeted them with a long-awaited hug. Despite the circumstances, it was a welcome reunion. The girls were comforted, and Midori was grateful that our family was finally all together in the same city to fight the battle ahead.

Chan had been like a member of the family since the kids were in middle school and was happy to help however she could. She stayed with the girls while they were in Honolulu, driving them wherever they needed to be, most often to the hospital. She helped lighten the mood with funny stories about life in Honolulu and reminisced with Dani, Jordan, and Scott about all the fun times we had shared over the years on Kauai. Like Midori and all the friends and family who would later visit, she weaved herself into our family and provided an extra source of strength for us to draw on during this inconceivable time.

Scott

Between the hospital and the hotel, Scott saw a couple across the street walking hand in hand. They were about our age, and he was struck by their peaceful demeanor. *Their lives are completely normal,* he thought, *just like our lives were just a few days ago.*

But now, here he was, on this side of the street, with his entire world turned upside down. His wife was on death's door, her body actively attacking itself, destroying her organs and killing her feet and hands. And here he was, on his way to deliver that dire news to our children.

When Scott arrived at the hotel, he found Chan, Jordan, and Dani strewn across one of the beds, telling stories like they used to when they were kids. He exchanged long hugs with them, feeling their trepidation as they anxiously awaited word of my condition.

He gently explained to the girls that I was sicker than expected. He confessed that the circulatory problems in my hands were serious and that my feet were beginning to show signs of similar damage. He relayed all of the information that the doctor and Maren had shared, their eyes growing wider and wetter as he spoke.

As hard as it was, he wanted to be honest with them. So he looked his daughters in the eyes and spoke words he never thought he'd have to say about their 52-year-old mother:

"The doctors are worried she might not make it through the night."

CHAPTER 8

SOMEWHERE BETWEEN LIFE AND DEATH

"Beginnings are usually scary, and endings are usually sad, but it's everything in between that makes it all worth living."

– Bob Marley

Tuesday, September 18 - Day Two in the ICU

Against all odds, I had made it through the first night in the Queen's ICU, a promising sign that my body was finding strength to fight the infection and ensuing sepsis. My medical team and family were overjoyed that I had gotten over this first hurdle. I was far from out of the woods, but they continued to focus on the positive and on the belief that I would recover.

Everyone was beginning to realize this would be a much longer and more involved process than any of them had imagined. They began preparing for a lengthy stay in Honolulu, focusing solely on the outcome that I would survive. It was clear I would have to recover on Oahu for a week or more before any possibility of transferring closer to family. Emotions had to be set aside as they managed the practical issues at hand.

They sent out a message asking if anyone had an Ohana unit (commonly called a mother-in-law unit on the mainland) or an apartment they could rent for a month. A friend of ours offered to lend my family a large condominium near the hospital. This was the perfect solution, as it would have room for the family and friends who would be visiting to help care for me when *(if!)* I woke up.

It was a blessing to have this beautiful home where Midori and my family could escape to get much-needed rest. Along with the hotel room in Waikiki, this kindness was just the beginning of the flood of gifts my family would receive to help us through this unprecedented time. Those gifts were a bright silver lining amid an otherwise awful experience.

Ashley & Ipo

Another stroke of luck: Joel's sister, Ashley, worked in social services at The Queen's Medical Center. She had been helping my family in any way she could since Sunday morning, when I was still on Kauai.

Ashley made a point of checking in on us often and arranged for Ipo, one of the hospital's trained support dogs, to visit the girls and Scott regularly, bringing them comfort as they sat by my side. Jordan described it in an update to family and friends, accompanied by a photo of Dani and her happily petting Ipo before visiting me in the ICU for the first time.

> "We met Ipo, the hospital therapy dog! (Thanks to Ashley!) We now have [Ipo's] information, so we can call her to come hang out with us whenever we need 😇."

The accompanying photo of Dani and Jordan sitting on the floor with a beautiful yellow Labrador lying between them is one of the most emotional photos I have from this time. For the few minutes that Ipo was with them, they were able to forget the dread they were feeling while I was on life support in the ICU.

Ipo and the other volunteer support dogs would later visit my family and me in my room. The amount of comfort this provided us cannot be overstated. In fact, at one point during my stay, the nurses put a sign on my door asking visitors not to disturb me while I was resting. Still, we didn't want to miss a visit from the support dogs, so Dani handwrote on the bottom of the sign, "EXCEPT DOGS! ALL DOGS WELCOME," so that they would be sure to stay or at least come back as soon as they could.

I can't say enough about the importance of having support animals in hospitals, nursing homes, schools, airports, courtrooms, or any other place where people need extra mental health support. I have since become an avid supporter of Assistance Dogs of Hawaii.[1] They provide people with disabilities professionally trained dogs that help increase their independence and enhance the quality of their lives. They are also committed to serving people with other special needs through their Facility Dog and Community Outreach Programs.

Dani & Jordan

As relieved as my daughters were that I had survived the night, seeing me in the ICU for the first time was shocking. I looked so swollen and helpless, like a shell of my former self. I had been healthy just a few days earlier and was now on mechanical ventilation, fighting for my life.

They sat by my side, each holding one of my hands as they comforted me with their voices. They wanted me to know I wasn't alone. They were there to support me. I was unable to respond, but they stayed by my side, telling me they knew I could get better and that all of our friends and family were praying for me. They listed the names of my extended family and best friends and reminded me of all of the people who loved me and were praying for me to live. Hoping that my unconscious brain was hearing some of their words,

---

1. Learn more: www.assistancedogshawaii.org

they wanted to remind me of all of the reasons I needed to fight to survive.

A Pressing Problem

As the hours and days passed in the ICU and I remained unconscious on the ventilator, my hands and feet became increasingly damaged from the DIC and vasopressors. Together, they were causing clotting and a reduction of much-needed blood flow to my dying hands and feet.

"We need to get her off these 'pressors," one of the nurses told Scott. This particular nurse was a favorite of his for her direct, no-nonsense communication style and high level of competence and care.

"Is she ready for that?" Scott asked the nurse, knowing she would be straight with him.

"There's only one way to find out," she told him. "I'm going to start reducing the dosage, and we'll watch how she responds."

Thankfully, my vitals continued to strengthen, and they were able to wean me off the vasopressors completely over the next 24 hours. Though this medication had helped save my life, it had also increased the damage to my hands and feet, so it was a tremendous relief to everyone when it was stopped.

"Katy Grainger Updates" Facebook Page

My family quickly became overwhelmed by the responsibility of making decisions for my care, the need to communicate with other family and close friends, and coordinating the logistics of an uncertain future. As much as they wanted to update all of our loved ones personally, they didn't have the energy to keep communicating with everyone individually, so they decided to set up a central communication system. This would allow them to streamline frequent updates to friends and family scattered across the United States.

The girls chose to start a private Facebook page for my health updates, since Facebook was where I had kept in touch with many of my friends and family on the mainland after we moved to Hawaii. They let everyone know about the new update page in texts and on my personal Facebook page and invited them to join if they were interested. Dani and Jordan managed the account, and Scott wrote medical updates for them to post daily.

Facebook update from Jordan:

> We have created this group to take some of the stress off of Midori, Dani and me. We are so grateful for the outpouring of love and support everyone has given Mom and us, but we figured it would be easier for everyone if we could just post the information we have here. If you have questions you're still welcome to reach out [phone numbers were provided]. You should be able to add people so you're welcome to add whoever wants to stay updated 🩶

I've since reviewed all of the updates and comments on my Facebook update page. From the very beginning, it's clear how quickly my tragic news spread within a concerned community. I saw the names of people I hadn't seen in years who began commenting while I was still in the ICU. They were commenting directly to my daughters and husband, wishing them well, offering prayers for a miraculous recovery, and letting them know they weren't alone during that scary time.

People shared stories of miraculous recoveries, touching quotes, beautiful photos, practical things like free air miles for travel, the names of specialists on the mainland, and housing that was available if we needed to fly to a hospital in a larger city where we didn't have connections.

The Facebook page served as a central hub where my friends and family could communicate about the situation. Our friends on Kauai arranged to take care of our home and watch our one-year-old puppy and elderly rescue dog while we were away. They used the

Facebook page to post regular photos of our dogs playing in the yard. Many people set up prayer groups within their faith communities and invited others to join.

Facebook update from Scott:[2]

> Katy is starting to stabilize, which is a good thing. Still some significant problems with fluid in lungs and circulation failure. Either of which has serious consequences if they deteriorate. / We are still well in the woods but she is making progress on her other symptoms: kidney failure and blood pressure. They should have some lab work back today that can give us specific pathogens to target with antibiotics. / Keep praying for her strength. We are all together (Midori, Scott, Dani, Jordan) on Oahu at Queens hospital holding mom's hand and passing on all your love.

Facebook was a place to share my condition from a perspective of faith and hope, but behind the scenes, my condition was often worse than Scott was willing to share beyond our inner circle.

Scott - text to close family:

> Katy's breathing tube is currently giving her 5x the oxygen that you and I breathe yet she is only actually getting 90% of the oxygen you and I get. This is really bad and must change and improve. It's a very big concern.

---

2. **DISCLAIMER:** Scott isn't a doctor so his medical explanations aren't 100% accurate. Always check with a doctor for medical questions and advice, and remember that every patient's experience is different.

> She also has bruising/purple discoloration in her hands and feet and a small bruising spot now appearing on her nose. This is a result of restricted blood flow due to the low blood pressure. There is also the possibility the restriction is caused by the infection releasing plaque in her vascular system which then flows to her capillaries in her hands and feet and clogs them [DIC]. This is also very concerning.

Wednesday, September 19 - ICU Day Three

I made it through a second night in the ICU, boosting my family's hope that I might have the strength to survive. But while recovery was looking increasingly possible, the damage to my hands and feet was looking increasingly catastrophic.

Facebook update from Dani:

> Dad, Jordan, Hunter, Midori and I are at the ICU with my mom now. Today's news on this recovery is both good and bad. The good news is that her BP is stabilized so she no longer requires medication [vasopressors]. The respiratory assistance with the breathing tube is being reduced and she is being weaned off of that. We also lowered her sedation momentarily so that we were able to talk to her. She opened her eyes a tiny bit and responded with movements to our voices. / A setback that was brought to our attention today is the capillary damage which occurred at the outset of her infection is worse than expected. We met with a vascular surgeon who said there is apparent damage due to lack of blood flow but recovery is possible. / Please please pray for vascular and circulatory healing in her hands and her feet. /

> Your prayers for getting her off of the blood pressure medicine and finding a home for us while we are here have been answered. Thank you all for your love and support. We can feel it all the way from here, and I'm sure Mom can as well.

If she survives...

While Scott and the girls were in the room with me, a young vascular surgeon came in to give Scott an update on my condition.

"A lot of times," he explained, "we can take an artery and bypass a clot, and that's how you can restore circulation. But in this case, the DIC has systemically clotted all of her capillaries. Think of it like a dry sponge: her capillaries aren't getting the blood flow they need to the soft tissues, and that's why she's got this gangrene in her hands and feet."

"So is it just her hands and feet that are affected?"

"No," the doctor replied, "DIC is systemic. It's impacting her whole body, including her vital organs."

That answer hit Scott like a ton of bricks, but he didn't want to press for more answers in front of the girls. Instead, he shifted back into problem-solving mode, thinking there might be restorative surgery that could be performed on my hands and feet, maybe a skin transplant of some kind?

"Okay, so what's the prognosis on her hands and feet?" Scott asked, expecting to hear a list of possible solutions.

"It's way too early to tell," said the doctor, shaking his head.

"Pretend it's not too early to tell," Scott insisted. "Just tell me what you think. I know you don't know for sure. I promise I won't hold you to it."

"Well," the doctor looked Scott directly in the eyes, "I think that, if she survives, she's likely to lose her hands above the wrists, and her feet below the knees."

Scott swallowed hard. "You mean… amputations?" It hadn't occurred to him before that moment that the only solution might be a permanent one.

The doctor nodded. "We might be able to save her hands. But her feet and fingertips? They're not going to recover."

Silence fell over the room as my husband and daughters confronted the reality of what I would be waking up to, if I woke up at all.

My family now understood that my extremities were not the only body parts that had been affected: I had also sustained damage to my kidneys, liver, lungs, heart, and likely my brain. To support these organs, I was placed on continuous kidney dialysis because my kidneys had failed. I still had a ventilator breathing for me. Blood was being drawn regularly to check the functioning of my weakening liver and heart. Every hour I survived and every tiny incremental improvement in my blood work improved my chances of survival.

Scott asked to speak to the doctors privately, away from the girls and me, so that he could ask them for a realistic assessment of my chances. One of my physicians explained that the top specialists in the hospital were attending to me as I was "the sickest person in the hospital." Since this was the only level-one trauma center in Hawaii, that likely made me the sickest hospitalized person in the entire state.

My ICU doctor then gently confirmed that if I did survive, Scott should expect that I would likely lose my hands and feet because of the blood clots and circulatory issues. He mentioned possible treatments (hyperbaric oxygen therapy and nitroglycerin cream), which might revive some of the flesh that was still viable. Still, he emphasized that these treatments weren't always successful and that my case was severe.

This was not the first time Scott had heard about these treatments. Julia's mother, Marnie, had been encouraging Scott to get me into a hyperbaric chamber as soon as possible. But since no machinery could accompany me into the chamber, I couldn't start those treatments until I was able to breathe independently.

But even in the face of this grim prognosis, Scott didn't give up hope. He posted requests on Facebook and texted family and close friends asking for prayers for continued improvements in my health, and special prayers for my hands and feet. We needed all the help we could get.

7:20 p.m. - Scott - text to a close friend:

Lock: What do we know Scotty?

Scott: Horrible complication surfaced today. She really needs your prayers.

There was forward progress coupled with a major setback. Progress on all recovery fronts: heart is good (low chance of endocarditis), lungs are improving, and she will go into interim dialysis (from full-time). All great.

Major setback: the infection attacked her microvascular (capillary) system at its outset. Forced the body to counter with microclots that lodged themselves in Katy's capillaries in hands and feet. Those capillary systems are now severely damaged. So blood circulation remains severely restricted even though the blood pressure meds were stopped super early. Micro-clots remain very problematic.

This is very, very serious and honestly terrifying me to the limit of my tolerance. However, we won't know how much permanent damage or amputation necessity for many weeks. So please pray for extensive vascular healing for her.

Scott was beginning to process that, even if I survived, our lives would be irreparably changed.

Accept the Help

That night, Dani reached out to Julia and shared the news that I might need amputations. Julia couldn't believe that the same condition that had ravaged her life, her body, and her family was now doing the same to my family and me. Imagine getting hit by lightning and finally recovering, then learning your best friend's mom has just been struck by lightning. As devastated as she was by the injustice of sepsis threatening my life and limbs, as it had done to her, she wanted to support Dani as much as possible.

Julia told Dani how sorry she was that our family was going through what her family had endured. Then she opened up and shared all the things she wished she and her family had known when she was fighting for her life and her limbs. She wanted to prepare Dani for the arduous journey ahead as best as she could.

In the best-case scenario, I would live, but my life would never be the same and neither would Dani's. Julia could tell that Dani was coming to terms with this reality, and she wanted to give her hope. She reassured her that I would adapt to whatever limb loss I experienced, just as she had. She reminded Dani of the support she would have from family and friends, and the fact that I was in the best place possible to get the care I needed.

"Your mom is going to be really confused when she wakes up," Julia warned. "She won't know what's going on, or what's happened to her body. You'll want to make her feel better, but you can't. There are a lot of things you won't be able to control. Focus on what you *can* do for her. Be there for her. Love her. Advocate for her. That's what my mom did for me. You're all going to have to do that for your mom. But you won't be doing it alone, my family is here to support you however we can, and so are so many other friends and family members. Accept all the help that's offered. You and your family don't need to go through this alone."

Thursday, September 20 - ICU Day Four

A New Hope

By now, word had spread about my condition. The diversity and number of friends joining the Facebook group, and the love, prayers, and support for my family and me in our greatest time of need, were overwhelming in the best way possible.

Text from my nephew Darrick to our family:

> The Facebook update page Dani and Jordan created has hundreds of close friends/family following, thousands of comments of love, support, and encouragement and arguably the best curated collection of dog photos on Facebook - it's uncanny how the worst of situations can bring out the best in people.

This incredible support helped bolster the spirits of Scott, Midori, and the girls as they trudged through the difficult days in the ICU, helplessly waiting for updates on my condition. The community encouragement made them feel less alone as they navigated the highs and lows of my daily medical reports.

#Katystrong

One of the sweetest gestures came from one of my best friends on Kauai. My friend Lisa ordered pink string "Katystrong" bracelets to wear in support of my family and me. What started as a small symbol of solidarity for friends on Kauai soon led to requests for bracelets from loved ones all over the country.

Lisa ended up sending hundreds of bracelets, in batches and individually, to my friends and family in other cities. She was ordering and sending bracelets for weeks. She later commented on how special it was to make personal connections with everyone who was praying for me and to have a way to help when she felt so helpless.

Dozens of friends and family members posted photos on my Facebook update page wearing the pink bracelets. Clearly, my story was impacting far more people than just me and my closest family.

Scott - text to close friends:

> The infectious disease specialist is still not able to locate the pathogen [causing the infection in Katy's body]. So we are continuing to use broad-spectrum antibiotics...

> Maren lands today. Love you guys! Keep us in your prayers!

Knowing Maren would be with Scott, the girls could take a break from the hospital as well. Scott felt it would be best for them to return to California for a few days for a previously planned trip to a friend's ranch for Dani's birthday. It would be good for them to get their minds off the helplessness of watching my body become so damaged from the sepsis and DIC.

He was concerned that when I was eventually brought out of my drug-induced coma, it might be difficult for me to breathe on my own. He didn't want the girls to witness that. But most of all, he didn't want them to have to see me realize how damaged my hands and feet had become. The ranch trip was a welcome excuse for them to give me a few days to get stronger before they saw me again.

They lowered my sedation that day, and Scott was able to ask me if I thought Jordan and Dani should leave me to celebrate Dani's birthday with her friends. We had talked about this trip before I became sick, and had both been excited for the girls to go to their friend's beautiful ranch. I nodded enthusiastically with my eyes closed and the breathing tube still in my throat.

As sick as I was, I had remembered the trip and wanted the girls to experience that special weekend with supportive friends. Scott was happy the girls knew they were leaving with my blessing. They were all relieved to see how well I seemed to understand what he was saying. This gave them hope that the sepsis hadn't damaged my brain.

I have seen this video many times. It warms my heart to know I was able to give my girls my blessing to take care of themselves in the midst of all that we were going through as a family.

Facebook update from Scott:

> Katy did her first interim [kidney] dialysis today. This is a big deal; it moved a lot of fluid in a relatively short 4hr time frame. Her success here helps remove fluid from her lungs and improves her respiratory function. / Goals of interim dialysis: 1) maintain blood pressure without BP enhancer meds, 2) remove fluid at a constant rate of removal (not too fast or too slow) and 3) remove 2 liters of fluid. She hit all 3 goals perfectly! Very happy about this. She does another tomorrow, then 3x/wk after that. Pray for consistency with her body response to the dialysis.

As my vital signs became stronger, my kidney dialysis was going well, and my bloodwork was showing improvement, my family's concern began to shift to my purple hands and feet, which were clearly dying from lack of oxygen.

Our limbs are so valuable to us. We use them all day, every day, to navigate our world. We even have an expression in English, "I would give an arm or leg to…" because giving up a limb symbolizes one of the most precious things a person can imagine losing.

This was the reality my family faced. Now that the odds of my survival were significantly improving, they were beginning to come to terms with the fact that my fingertips and toes wouldn't be saved, and began to imagine a future for me where I might not have hands or feet at all. They believed I could find happiness in that future, but continued to hold out hope for a miracle.

Scott tried to keep the Facebook posts hopeful but was more

unguarded with close friends and family. One of our best friends asked how he was doing.

"Hardest thing I've ever experienced," was his reply.

He soldiered on and continued to communicate with my medical team while translating all he learned into texts to family and daily Facebook updates.

Friday, September 21 - ICU Day Five

Changing of the Guard

Facebook update from Midori:

> I was reading articles from the Goop blog to Katy and after about an hour I said… "Are you tired of hearing my voice. Should I stop?" and she shook her head NO several times! Happy, happy! If anyone has any articles that you think Katy would like, please post the links and we can read them to her!

The improvements in my health and the impending arrival of Maren allowed Midori to return to Seattle to be there for her elderly mother, who had been in poor health for some time. Midori's brother had called the night before with dire news: their mom was in the hospital again, this time with pneumonia and, of all things, sepsis.

The confirmation that I was aware of what was going on around me and had heard everything she'd said to me was a massive relief to Midori. It felt like a sign that I was going to be okay and she could safely leave to be with her family.

As suggested reading materials poured in on the Facebook comments, Midori read me the articles, making sure to tell me who suggested them and reminding me how much these people meant to me and I to them. She was happy to have this quality time with me before she had to return home.

Maren

Facebook update from Scott:

> Today was a good day. Maren (Scott's MD sister-in-law) arrived from Palo Alto and will help comfort Katy, advocate for Katy's care and support Scott. Katy did a 30-minute trial breathing tube removal (extubation). Did very well. / She's still not quite ready to breathe completely on her own so it will be another day or so before the extubation. But real progress. She also is communicating with us. Nodding or shaking her head to yes/no answers. That's wonderful and exciting. Her kidneys are still shut down so she does dialysis 3x/wk. her first [interim] treatment yesterday went really well. / Pray for continued improvement in Katy's kidneys [and that] she remains stable. The microclots in her capillaries remain very problematic. Please continue to pray to improve Katy's blood flow to her extremities. But overall a good day today.

Maren's arrival in Honolulu was a relief to everyone. The girls and Midori were comforted that a close family member with critical medical knowledge would be with Scott in their absence, especially when I made the difficult transition to breathing independently.

Maren took the night shift by my side so that Scott could go to the condo and get some much-needed rest. Unfortunately, he still wasn't able to sleep because he was worried about all the things that could go wrong the next day when the breathing tube would be removed from my throat.

He tried to meditate to calm his mind, but the intrusive thoughts were relentless. He finally drifted off to sleep but was awakened by a nightmare in which I couldn't see anything after coming out of the coma. He remembered hearing somewhere that becoming blind after septic shock and DIC was a possibility.

He texted Maren in a panic in the middle of the night, asking if I could be blind. She was sleeping and never responded. He searched the internet and read academic articles and stories of other sepsis survivors, which only fueled his worries.

He'd been mentally rehearsing what he would say to me when I woke up and saw the state of my hands and feet. What he'd settled on was, "You can still hold your grandchildren, even without hands."

But what if she can't see those grandchildren? Then what will I tell her?

Struggling to Survive

My week in the ICU was a blur, not just for me but for my friends and family. They sat by my side as a machine breathed for me, and a complex array of tubes and wires entwined my body, delivering medications and monitoring my vital signs: heart rate, breathing, oxygen levels, temperature, and blood pressure. They watched helplessly as my fingertips turned from plum to eggplant to black, and the maroon spots on my hands wove together up to my wrists. My feet, which showed minimal damage when I arrived at Queen's, had now turned a sickly purplish-red as well. Even my nose and cheeks started to look bruised due to lack of oxygen.

The strength displayed by Scott and my daughters, with the help of Midori and other friends and family, was nothing short of heroic. The outpouring of love and support from our extended community was astounding. It was a testament to how people come together to support someone in crisis.

CHAPTER 9

AWAKENING TO A NEW REALITY

" 'It seems very pretty,' she said when she had finished it, 'but it's rather hard to understand!' (You see, she didn't like to confess, even to herself, that she couldn't make it out at all.) 'Somehow it seems to fill my head with ideas – only I don't know exactly what they are! However, somebody killed something: that's clear, at any rate.' "

– Alice, *Alice Through the Looking Glass*

Saturday, September 22 - First Day Awake in ICU

Back to Life

September 22nd was the day I was reborn into a new reality. I remember a few parts of it clearly, but most of the next eight days were shrouded in a fog of confusion and fear called Post-ICU delirium (also called ICU delirium or just delirium). My memories of that time are a swirl of uncertainty, starting with moments of clarity, going in and out of sleep, hallucinating, and experiencing the worst nightmares of my life, not knowing what was real and what was a dream.

Facebook update from Scott:

> Katy had a successful extubation today. She is now breathing with only oxygen mask assistance. Huge step! Prayers her lungs continue to clear up and improve to where she can breathe without assistance. / Dani and Jordan returned to California yesterday and sent a video to Mom today on Dani's birthday. She smiled and nodded. Yes yes yes the whole way through. Incredible. Her hands and feet still remain critical but we believe they are showing improvement as well. / Continue focused prayer on healing the capillaries in her hands and feet and removing the microclots from them. On this long road to Katy's recovery, today has been a good day. Hold on to it and pray for another one for her tomorrow.

It began with a nurse's voice waking me up, saying loudly, "Katy, you are in the hospital. You have been very sick. You have a tube in your throat that's helping you breathe. I'm going to remove it now so you can breathe on your own. On the count of three, I want you to cough, and I will pull the tube out of your throat."

And then, quicker than I expected, she counted, "One, two, three."

I obediently coughed, expecting the tube to magically disappear. Instead, I gagged violently as the nurse pulled out the impossibly long tube. My throat hurt, as if I had been choked, and I could taste something bitter in my mouth. I was struggling to breathe and trying not to vomit from the discomfort and repulsive taste as the tube passed painfully through my throat and mouth.

My eyes opened suddenly, only to be blinded by a bright light shining down on me. I squinted as Scott's blurry face came into view from the side. He brought his face close to mine like he had when I'd given birth to both of our daughters. He held my face in his hands, directing me to look at him.

"Can you see me?" he asked anxiously.

"No," I croaked, distracted by the bright light as I groggily blinked, trying to adjust my eyes.

"Can you see the light?" he asked.

"No," I responded again, unclear of what I was saying and feeling disoriented.

I felt paranoid, like Scott was blocking my view of something he didn't want me to see. I wanted him to move out of the way so I could see where I was and figure out what was happening. I was unsettled and scared. I had no comprehension of what was going on, just a gut feeling that something was seriously wrong. My eyes darted all over the room, unable to focus on anything.

He backed away so the nurses could remove the monitoring tubes and cables. As my arms were lifted so that a cord could be freed from beneath them, I saw that there was something black on the tips of each of my fingers, like pen caps, and that my fingers and hands were an unnatural reddish-purple, as if I were wearing gloves.

Why am I wearing gloves in Hawaii?

As I strained to figure out what I was looking at, I noticed that the shrunken black things on my fingers had opaque fingernails on them with long white tips. They looked like the fingers of a storybook witch or something out of a zombie movie. I couldn't grasp what I was seeing.

Then the horror began to sink in.

These black things ARE *my fingertips! That red-violet color is my* SKIN*!*

A knot formed in my stomach that would be with me for weeks. Despair took hold of me as I tried to make sense of why I was in the hospital and what had happened to my hands.

I was more afraid than I had ever been in my life. Though I couldn't get a grasp on what it was, I knew something tragic had happened that neither of us could undo.

The drugs coursing through my body took me in and out of mental clarity. I felt the room distorting around me like a psychedelic drug trip in a movie. The lights, the nurses, and Scott were all circling my bed in a chaotic swirl. When I closed my eyes, I kept seeing my fingertips, blackened and shriveled, swimming around me like a school of monstrous fish. These hallucinations would haunt me for the next week as I came in and out of awareness.

Between the crazy doom visions that were running through my mind and a general state of disorientation and delusion, I was trying to process what could have happened to my fingers. I felt paranoid and began worrying about what could have happened to the rest of my body.

Scott kept trying to get my attention as he held my hand, rubbing the back of it with his thumb. He looked at me anxiously, almost desperately. A sparkling film of tears reflected in his red-rimmed eyes.

He always had the most beautiful blue eyes. They had caught my attention when I first saw him at 15 and they continued to mesmerize me for more than 35 years.

His eyes took me out of my chaotic mind for a minute and made me feel safe, as they always had.

But they looked so sad.

What is happening??

"You can't see anything at all?" He asked with urgency.

"Yes," I croaked, feeling annoyed by the brightness of the room. "There's a really bright light. I can't see anything because it's shining in my eyes."

He moved his face even closer to mine, blocking the light with his head.

"Can you see me now?" he asked frantically.

"Yes," I said, irritated and confused. My brain was straining to make sense of what I was seeing. My thoughts were fractured by shock, disorientation, and the many drugs that were still impacting my body.

Having Scott with me eased my paranoia. I felt protected with him there. I saw the man I had loved since high school, and knew I wasn't in this horrible situation alone. I was grateful to see him, but my emotions were all over the place. One minute, I was sure we could get through anything together, but the next minute my thoughts would slip back to my black fingertips. I would become confused, distraught, and afraid once again.

How did this happen?!

The only things I could recall during my time at Wilcox were the oozing sore on my thumb and breathing through an oxygen mask. Questions were swirling through my clouded brain.

How did this make me so sick? Why am I so out of it? Is my brain damaged? Am I dying? What else is wrong with me?

At some point later that day, I came to realize it wasn't just my fingertips that were affected. My feet had circulatory problems as well. Scott told me about the damage when I asked him what else had happened to me.

I immediately asked to see them. He gently pulled back my blankets, revealing my unnaturally pale, skinny legs and liver-colored feet. I was stunned. The color was much darker than my hands. My toes were pointed away from my body and appeared to be as black as my fingertips.

My right ankle throbbed with pain, and both feet felt like they were being crushed under something heavy or forced into too-small boots. I made Scott keep my feet out of the blankets when he pulled them back up to my waist in hopes that it would hurt less. Even the gentle weight of the bedcovers seemed heavy on them. Unfortunately, it didn't relieve the pain. Nothing did.

I tried to move my feet, but couldn't. That was too much for me to handle, so my mind conveniently locked all of the information about them in a vault to deal with later.

In order to give my body every chance to heal, I needed to hold on to hope for as long as I could. It's amazing to look back and realize how my mind was protecting me from the things I wasn't ready to process.

Post-ICU Delirium

Scott - text to our extended family:

> Another major challenge at this stage is post-ICU delirium. Basically, temporary brain damage caused by the event coupled with the surreal life confined to the 24/7 ICU madhouse. She has many delusions about events that didn't happen, things going to happen that aren't, conspiracies, paranoia and insomnia.

> It is transitory but WOW is it challenging! I would really like this whole phase to end now.

> Please pray for continued recovery, calm, trust, courage, peace and light for Katy. Overall her recovery progresses every day and it is a miracle she is alive. Love u guys. Grainger ohana.

Looking back now, I realize my fractured thoughts were delusional hallucinations that began as soon as I was awakened in the ICU. They came and went throughout the day and got worse at night.

The frequent and varied exams I underwent in the ICU were translated into horrific assaults in my muddled memory, and my family endured the same looping conversation again and again. They would patiently listen as I repeatedly described all the terrible things I believed I was experiencing, then gently but firmly reassure me that I had not been left alone for even a moment during my hospital stay, nor would I ever be left alone for any reason. Sadly, this only served to convince me that it was a conspiracy they were all in on and that no one around me could be trusted.

After all, part of my body had died, and nobody was talking about that. I had seen my black fingertips and instinctively knew they couldn't be saved, but nobody was acknowledging it. What other horrors were they keeping from me? What else was dead and gone?

Meanwhile, when I closed my eyes to try to sleep, loud dance music was playing in my head at a volume you would hear in a club. The only thing that would make the music stop was opening my eyes, but that was difficult, and the music was too loud for me to sleep. I was exhausted.

In hindsight, it's possible I was sleeping the whole time and dreamt it all. Regardless, it interfered with the rest I needed to regain my strength. I'll never actually know what was real and what was a dream or hallucination. What I do know now is that it was all caused by post-ICU delirium. It was one of the worst nights of my life.

As if I Wasn't Going Through Enough

For some awful reason, soon after I was extubated, my brain created a horrific scenario – one of the worst things I could imagine. In trying to make sense of what had happened to me, and the horrible feeling of dread that wouldn't go away, I came to believe I had been in an accident with one of my daughters and she had not survived.

I was too afraid to ask about it. Afraid they wouldn't tell me the truth, and even more afraid it might be true. So I sat silent and alone in my terror and despair until I fell back to sleep.

When I awoke, I was disoriented and once again had no idea what had happened. Scott kept mentioning Midori, Dani, and Jordan, saying they had been with me "all week" in the hospital and were so relieved to know I was awake and doing well. But in my mind, I'd seen them just a few days before – in California!

I argued with him and told him they hadn't been in Hawaii. I believed it was still the prior Sunday. I was struggling to understand why he was in the hospital with me when I had just been exchanging texts with him on his fishing trip in Idaho. He tried to explain that I had been sleeping for almost a week and that Midori and our daughters had arrived when I was unconscious. I had the hardest time understanding this. It made no sense that they would come all this way when we had just been together so recently.

Then I remembered something about one of the girls being hurt. *Is she okay? Where is she? Is she in the hospital too?* I couldn't allow myself to think about it and I was still too scared to ask.

This confusion began a cycle of paranoia, feeling like Scott was keeping things from me. It only made it worse when the hospital staff would try to help him explain it to me, because then I felt like they were all in on the conspiracy.

I had no understanding of what I had been through in the last week, how sick I had been, and how close I had come to dying. I would forget that something may have happened to one of my daughters, but then I would remember and feel miserable all over again.

When I wasn't worrying about them, I was grateful my girls weren't there to see me like that. I knew my body was in bad shape. I was told I needed kidney dialysis. I worried I might need a kidney transplant, or dialysis for the rest of my life, or might even have a colostomy bag. That was never a possibility for me, but it seemed plausible in my paranoid state.

Later in the day, Scott showed me videos of the girls, proving once and for all that they were both alive and well and enjoying the trip they had been planning when we were together in California. I remembered them preparing for that trip. I was overjoyed to see videos of their weekend with friends and farm animals, realizing they were both safe. It was thrilling to hear them tell me how happy they were to see me awake and that they couldn't wait to come visit me again.

Dani text to Maren (with us in Honolulu):

> Tell my mom talking to her was the best birthday present and I love her so much

Scott text to extended family:

> Just shared with Katy pictures and videos of Dani and Jordan this wknd at a ranch. She's making small complete sentences. She was in a coma three hours ago. So that's amazing.

> THEN she asked Maren when she was leaving. Maren said in two days. Katy says, "On Monday?" Maren says, "How'd you know that!?!" Katy: "Well I know today's Saturday, Dani's birthday!" Right now she's listening to Jordan's laugh on the video over and over... so incredible!!

Dream Team

Despite these challenges, I soon became energized by the excitement of my family and medical team. Scott was clearly relieved I was breathing on my own and able to interact with everyone. Every doctor and nurse who entered my room smiled from ear to ear and said how happy they were to see me awake and alert, interacting appropriately. I could understand them and answer questions. I finally made sense when I spoke. That meant that in addition to breathing on my own, I appeared to be hearing and seeing. I was now reasoning clearly between the bouts of post-ICU delirium.

After one of several naps, I awoke in my hospital room to the sight of a young doctor standing at the foot of my bed. He had bright eyes, crinkled at the edges by his enormous smile. I assumed I must have known him by the way he was grinning at me. I smiled back, hoping he would remind me who he was.

He exclaimed, "I cannot believe how good you look!"

Embarrassed, I thought, *Oh my gosh, I must look so beautiful right now!*

Before I could sort out what was happening, he went on.

"You know, we weren't sure we would ever see you with your eyes open. You were very sick. You look so healthy! Nothing at all like the woman I saw in the ICU. I just can't get over how good you look right now!"

That was quite the welcome back into the world. I'd already realized what a miracle it was that I was alive when I saw the tears in my husband's eyes as I recognized his face, but now I was beginning to understand that I had been given a second chance at life.

The young doctor asked me a few questions to see how clearly I was thinking, despite my disorientation.

"Do you know the date?"

"September twenty-second," I proudly replied, recalling Scott telling me earlier that it was my daughter's birthday. It felt like I was cheating because it was a date I knew so well.

"Do you know where you are?"

"Yes, Queen's Hospital." Someone must have told me that earlier too.

"The Queen's Medical Center! Yes, that's exactly where you are."

Then he threw me a curveball. "Do you know what city you're in?"

I thought about it for a minute. I had no idea what city I was in, but I was trying to put it together using context clues. I knew I'd gotten sick on Kauai, which is in the middle of the Pacific Ocean. I tried to imagine the location of the biggest and best hospital they would have transported me to.

Having just met a nurse who was originally from Manila, I guessed. "The Philippines?"

He laughed and said, "No, you're in Honolulu. It's a good thing you're not in the Philippines; that's a long way from here. You wouldn't have survived the trip!"

I felt embarrassed by my confusion, but buoyed by his excitement. I still remember that conversation like it was yesterday. It was the moment I became fully aware that I had survived something catastrophic and was surrounded by people who were incredibly grateful to see me alive.

Scott had been sharing messages with me all day. In addition to the videos and texts from the girls, all my closest friends and family were reaching out, excited that I was doing so well. Their enthusiasm helped ground me, and I was able to revel in my survival and set aside concern about my hands and feet.

The moment I fell asleep, though, the delusions returned. Most were terrifying, but after the fabulous meeting with my smiling doctor, I had one singularly lovely dream that still makes me smile when I think of it.

I dreamt I was in the hospital, working out with an ICU nurse. Scott and I were in a physical therapy room lifting weights. I was wearing a cute Lululemon outfit. My body was healthy, like it had been before I got sepsis, and everyone was impressed with me.

They applauded, saying, "We can't believe you're winning this competition," with the same infectious enthusiasm my doctor had shown earlier.

Scott cheered me on while showing me how to take deep breaths. "You're doing a great job," he told me. "You're winning!"

I believed him. I felt like a winner.

My doctors and other nurses suddenly appeared and chimed in, "You're the best we've ever seen! No one has ever done as well as you!"

I was so proud seeing everyone smiling and applauding for me. It felt like I was standing on a podium in a stadium with flowers and crowds cheering as if I had just won an Olympic medal.

I beat impossible odds that day, and was supported and loved. That was how my medical team and family made me feel. Even after waking up from that dream, that sense of pride stayed with me. I knew I had accomplished something tremendous, and everyone around me knew it too. I took that feeling of being supported and loved into the following days, weeks, months, and years of my recovery.

CHAPTER 10

BUILDING A WINNING TEAM

"One thing about championship teams is that they're resilient. No matter what is thrown at them, no matter how deep the hole, they find a way to bounce back and overcome adversity."

– Nick Saban

Standing By

Since I was expected to be at The Queen's Medical Center for at least three to four more weeks, my family began making plans for additional support. They wanted me to have close friends and family nearby at all times.

Scott knew he couldn't do it alone. He was exhausted from learning everything he could about my condition, interfacing with doctors, and writing daily Facebook updates for family and friends, all while emotionally supporting me and our girls. He was burning himself out.

To give everyone time away from the hospital, my core team divided the day into three eight-hour shifts. One person was assigned to be with me during each shift so the others could get away to rest, exercise, and have time to themselves while ensuring I was never left alone. By prioritizing their wellness, they were able to support mine without burning out.

Having my best friends and closest family with me every day meant I was never by myself in the room, and Scott and Dani could take breaks as needed. This strategy of 24-hour coverage made me feel safe as I grappled with my tremendous loss. It also ensured that someone was always available to speak with my medical team during their rounds. I was on painkillers, sick and weak, and not emotionally or mentally able to manage my own care in any way.

In addition to the friends who visited, receiving daily messages from people who couldn't be there reminded me that a supportive community surrounded me. Everyone who reached out made it clear they would be with me as long as I needed them. I felt reassured by their loving care.

While Scott was away from the hospital, the girls bought a notebook at the gift shop and left it in my room so no medical details would be missed. My caregivers used it to take notes on relevant details of my day and meetings with my medical team, which helped all of my supporters stay up to date on my condition. It also allowed Scott to step away without feeling like he would miss something important.

Having loved ones nearby empowered me to focus solely on allowing my body to heal and gain strength. Whenever I openly worried about my future or got frustrated with how slowly I was healing, they would assure me they had everything under control and encourage me to be patient, reminding me of how happy they were that I was alive and doing so well. This constant affirmation of their love and support let me know I wasn't in this battle alone.

I genuinely believe that if my family had not been there helping me through these first few days, I would have been too tired to increase my oxygen levels and clear my lungs, and I likely would not have survived.

Dani and Jordan

Dani extended her leave from work and committed to being with us throughout my hospital stay. Her employer was understanding and assured her she would be welcomed back whenever she was ready to return.

Dani was, in many ways, an ideal caregiver. She was gentle and nurturing, as well as methodical and diplomatic. She rose to the occasion and became my biggest cheerleader, helping her dad support me, manage the many people assisting us, and make sure I had everything I needed. Her calming presence, along with her undying support, was invaluable to me and everyone involved in my care. I came to rely on her almost as much as I relied on Scott.

At first, Jordan had told Scott she wanted to take a year off from school to stay by my side, missing out on the year abroad in Rome she'd been so looking forward to. But Scott set her straight.

"This is your Mom," he reminded her. "More than anything, she wants you to have a great life. Dropping out of school and missing out on the opportunity of a lifetime to be at her bedside 24/7 is not her idea of a great life for you. The best gift you can offer her is to go out there and live the most incredible life you can and be the amazing person she knows you can be."

Reluctantly, Jordan agreed to stay in school with the understanding that she could help by managing the Facebook updates and communicating with the family and me daily. She also worked with Dani and Midori to reach out to friends and family who had volunteered to help. She asked them to schedule flights to Honolulu in three-to-four-day shifts to spend time with me while I was at Queen's. We soon had more volunteers than we needed.

Jordan hated being so far away, but she understood that we wanted her to stay on track to graduate on time with her friends the following year. She knew we had enough people to help in the hospital, which allowed her to focus on school.

Jordan texted regularly and spoke with Scott and Dani in the early days, when my voice was too weak to talk on the phone. She made me daily videos while walking home from class or getting ready for sorority events, so I could watch them when I wasn't sleeping or seeing specialists. I have dozens of videos she sent me. They were an ideal way to communicate with me at that time. I still watch them occasionally when I need a little pick-me-up because they never fail to remind me of how loved and supported I was and still am.

Both girls were learning, along with the rest of us, the importance of asking for and accepting help when needed, as well as being able to pivot: shifting priorities to accommodate unexpected events.

Hunter and Kai

We were grateful that, in addition to supportive friends, both Dani and Jordan had loving partners to help them through this trying time. Both young men rose to the occasion by walking alongside the girls and our family as we navigated this grueling journey.

Hunter, Dani's boyfriend since her sophomore year of high school, lived on the Big Island, a 45-minute flight away from Honolulu. He joined our family on my second day in the ICU and continued to visit throughout my recovery. Having him there was a tremendous source of support for all of us. He'd been part of our family for years, and his bright, charming personality was a comfort to everyone.

Jordan's boyfriend, Kai, was one of Hunter's and Dani's best friends. They began dating over the summer, while Jordan was working in Los Angeles and Kai was starting his career near Santa Barbara. My illness presented a challenge at the beginning of their relationship. Still, Kai rose to the occasion, driving three hours through heavy traffic nearly every weekend to support Jordan through this difficult time while she remained at school. Scott and I were comforted throughout my recovery, knowing that our girls had this remarkable love and support in their lives.

Maren - My Sister-in-Law

Facebook update from Scott:

> Aunt Maren has been incredible at the hospital and has been helping Katy and Scott understand what's going on and keeping them calm with the whole situation.

My first night after I woke up in the ICU was extremely difficult. I remember waking up in a dark room, confused and disoriented, in severe pain. My right ankle and both feet were throbbing, my throat hurt, my whole body ached, and I felt nauseated, weak, and shaky.

The room was cold, and a humming sound and glowing lights emanated from unknown medical monitors. I could hear people in the hall and see light coming from under a distant door. I tried to raise myself in bed but couldn't. Cords tethered me uncomfortably to the mysterious machines surrounding my bed. I didn't know how to reach a nurse.

Seeing that Maren was there with me, I tried to say her name. My voice was barely audible and she was asleep, so she didn't hear me. I tried saying it louder, but my voice was too weak to wake her.

Then, in a surprising moment of clarity, I remembered hearing somewhere that if you yell "Mom" in a crowd, all mothers will instinctively pay attention. So, the third time, instead of saying "Maren," I took as deep a breath as I could with my weak lungs and squeaked the word "Mom!"

It worked! She woke up immediately and came to my bedside. I told her I was in pain, so she found a nurse who administered medications to make me more comfortable. I was too agitated and afraid to sleep because of delusions, nightmares, and a foreboding sense that I would never be the same healthy person I had been before.

Neither Maren nor I got much rest that night. She stayed awake with me to ensure I was getting the care I needed and to help calm my fears. I felt helpless and afraid I might stop breathing if I fell asleep, but having her there made me feel safer.

Sunday Morning, September 23 - Maren - text to extended family:

> Last night was a tough night for Katy, but she's so much better today! Doing breathing exercises with Scott. He's got a superpower when it comes to motivational training. Must have been all the soccer coaching. If she does her breathing exercises, they will be able to get her in the hyperbaric chamber to help her hands and feet later this week. So, exciting news!

My body was still weak, and my lungs were infiltrated with fluid, making it difficult to absorb oxygen. They were concerned that if my oxygen levels got too low, I might need to be placed back on mechanical ventilation, which would put me at risk for pneumonia and delay treatment for my dying limbs.

Scott later filled supporters in on details about the challenges facing me in the first days as I began breathing on my own.

Sunday Night, September 23 - Facebook update from Scott:

> Sunday was a day of prayer. [It] was also a day of remarkable turnaround and progress for Katy.... / [Katy's] turnaround followed a very difficult Saturday night. Fluid returned to her lungs and she was very close to pneumonia, which would require re-intubation, a potentially devastating setback. She hovered at the minimum O2 threshold most of the night. Extremely stressful. / She worked nonstop throughout the day. She progressed so far in 10 hours she now meets the respiratory threshold that would allow her to leave ICU!

Having helped us through the most challenging days of my recovery, Maren had to return to work. Before she left, she warned Scott that the next few days could be difficult as the ICU doctors were trying to balance my pain medications while not interfering with my reflex to breathe. She wanted him to understand that this was not unusual and that the medical team there was trained to help patients regain the ability to breathe on their own after mechanical ventilation. They were both comforted knowing that Holly was coming to take Maren's place.

Holly - My Sister-in-Law

Monday Morning, September 24 - Facebook update from Scott:

> Intensivist just came to our room. Katy has been downgraded. Her respiratory condition is stable but needs to improve. Her kidneys have begun to barely function but are moving [in the] right direction. BP solid. Hands and feet still really damaged but not getting worse. So they just downgraded her to stable and will soon be getting her out of ICU! This is great news.

Holly arrived on Monday, just as Maren was leaving. Her first shift was challenging because of my unstable health and the many appointments that filled my days.

I still had severe ICU delirium and was confused about why I was in the hospital. I couldn't understand why Maren had come to Hawaii for so short a time and was already leaving. Usually, when we had guests from the mainland, they stayed for at least a week and planned their trips well ahead of time. Why were she and Holly suddenly there with no warning? I was happy to see them, but in my disoriented state, I felt like I was failing as a hostess. I had to be constantly reminded that everyone was there to take care of me, not the other way around.

Every Breath I Took

I clearly remember Scott and Holly waking me up regularly and making me do breathing exercises when my oxygen levels would drop because of the medications I was taking. I later learned that they would watch my levels on the monitors while I slept, waking me when the numbers dipped to help me get more oxygen in my lungs so I wouldn't need to be reintubated and could start the hyperbaric treatments they hoped would save my limbs.

At the time, I was angry at being woken up so often by Scott and Holly. I knew they knew it, but they kept doing it anyway, which made me even more furious. I remember Scott standing in front of me, demonstrating what he wanted me to do by sucking in a deep breath and holding it for what seemed like an impossibly long time, then blowing it out.

I hated it when he asked me to breathe with him. I was exhausted, and it was hard for me to breathe so deeply. Undaunted by my annoyance, knowing it was the only thing he could do to help me heal, Scott continued to show me how to increase the vitally important oxygen in my blood. I knew my anger at his efforts was misplaced, but I couldn't help my sleep-deprived reaction.

"Where did you learn how to do this?" I remember asking him. Despite my exhaustion and annoyance, I couldn't help but be impressed with his expertise.

"Coaching Soccer," he told me, explaining that breathing was an essential part of the training regimen he'd used to coach girls' high school soccer over the past few years. When I copied his deep breaths, he showed me on the monitors that my blood oxygen levels would rise.

"How do you know what all those numbers on the monitors mean?" I was amazed by his understanding of what looked like random digits on a screen. In addition to my oxygen levels, he was able to tell me about all of my vital signs at a glance.

A nurse who was in the room at the time reminded me that Scott had been in the hospital with me since I got there a week earlier, and had been learning everything he could about my treatment so he could help me recover. Her tone conveyed admiration and appreciation for his diligence.

I felt embarrassed, as if I'd just asked an obvious question about a movie I'd fallen asleep in the middle of. I had slept through the past week and had no sense of time. I felt like I was still in the Kauai hospital with some sort of flu.

When Scott left to get some rest, the job of breathing coach fell to Holly, one of the most caring people I know. I thought the breathing exercises would stop when Scott left; I couldn't believe Holly was making me do them too! It's the only time in my life I can recall being upset with Holly Grainger.

When I begged her to stop, she patiently explained why we had to do this: if my oxygen levels dropped to the 92% range, an alarm would trigger, and the nurse would come in. If that happened, there was a chance I would have to be put back on a ventilator.

That got my attention. I couldn't remember being on the ventilator, but I recalled with painful clarity the bitter choking as it was pulled out of my throat. I never wanted to go through that again.

She pointed out the numbers on my monitors that showed my oxygen saturation and made a game out of taking deep breaths to slowly increase the number on the monitor by one percentage point at a time. If I took a deep enough breath and held it for a few seconds, we could sometimes increase the number by one percent in just one breath. Making it into a game made it much easier and more enjoyable for me, and I knew that when I got the number up to 99%, she'd let me go back to sleep.

Looking back, I now realize that every time Scott, Holly, or anybody else woke me up and asked me to breathe or to blow into the device that would strengthen my lungs and help me clear out the fluids, they were saving my life. I think of this often and have such gratitude that, despite my resistance, they literally helped me breathe to stay alive.

Tuesday Evening, September 25 - Facebook update from Scott:

> Tuesday was a busy day for Katy. Besides her daily regimen of specialist consults, X-rays, medicine regimen and examinations, she had physical therapy, a main catheter replacement (minor surgery) and dialyses. Very full day.... / Katy's recovery now focuses on 1) no major setbacks: lung fluid (pneumonia) and secondary infection (a repeat of sepsis event) are concerns here. However, each day of progression lowers the risk of these significantly. 2) Katy's healing also really focusing now on freeing the microclots in her capillaries to allow continued blood flow and healing of her liver, hands, and feet. 3) Emotional healing and restoration of Katy's energy.

Scott and Holly's hard work with those breathing exercises paid off when they got the news that my lungs were clearing and I could soon be moved out of the ICU. That meant I would be able to go into the hyperbaric chamber, which could help save my hands and feet.

Life in the ICU is full of second guessing and fear. Even though this was the news they wanted to hear, Scott worried they might be rushing my release. He was afraid I could relapse and end up getting sicker.

He called Maren, who assured him there was a stringent protocol for releasing me, and it was good news that I met their criteria. Being released from the ICU meant I was strong enough to go into the hyperbaric chambers that might help save my hands and feet from the vascular damage caused by the vasopressors and DIC. She knew better than any of us that I needed all available treatments as quickly as possible, if there was any chance of saving my damaged limbs.

She also reminded him regularly how essential it was that I be given the time and space I needed to make sense of my situation and come to my own conclusions. Having done a lot of work in patient advocacy and end-of-life care, Maren understood that denial was a natural part of my process and acceptance could not be rushed or forced upon me. Though Scott and my other supporters were with me on this journey, at the end of the day, it was my journey to navigate in my own time and my own way.

Teamwork Makes the Dream Work

Building a winning recovery team isn't just about getting the most qualified medical professionals on board. It's about ensuring everyone works together as a cohesive unit, with the sole purpose of doing everything they can to support the patient's best interests, emotionally, mentally, and physically.

Everyone who wants to support you should do their best to understand your medical condition, what you need, when you need it, and how best to provide it to you. Being surrounded by loving support isn't just helpful in a practical sense. It's what gives a patient hope and motivates them to keep on trudging through the darkness.

CHAPTER 11

FINDING FAITH IN THE DARKNESS

"To live without hope is to cease to live."

– Fyodor Dostoyevsky

God, grant me...

Up to this point, I haven't mentioned Scott's or my sobriety. But it feels important to share here because it was the first time we faced significant challenges as a married couple and learned how to get through difficult times together. It was a complicated dynamic that I'll simplify to give a bit of insight into how we became the people we were when I got sepsis.

I quit drinking in college because of alcoholism in my family, but Scott continued to drink, mostly socially, until our kids were born. We were in our early 30's then. He was trying to manage the pressure of supporting our young family financially, while I had left my career behind to become a stay-at-home mom.

I loved being with the kids, but managing the household didn't come naturally to me, so evenings were chaotic as we scrambled to figure out dinners and clean up the day's messes. To cope with the chaos at home and the stress of his job, Scott began working longer hours and drinking more. Meanwhile, I became increasingly resentful, overwhelmed, and frustrated with my inability to get on top of my tasks. We were under a lot of stress, and neither of us was coping well.

The pressure was tearing us apart. We knew we loved each other and our children more than anything, and we wanted our marriage to succeed, but we felt helpless to find a solution.

That helplessness, and our willingness to admit it, is what saved our marriage. We pulled together as a team and committed to finding the resources we needed. In our research, we found the Serenity Prayer by Reinhold Niebuhr and took it to heart: *God grant me the serenity to accept the things I cannot change, the courage to change the things I can, and the wisdom to know the difference.* Together, we found the courage to change what we could to get our family life back on track.

Over several difficult months, with guidance and hard work, along with the resulting lifestyle changes, we each found healthy coping strategies and recommitted to one another and our marriage. It was a difficult season, but it renewed our faith in God and community, strengthened our bond, and helped us prioritize family above all else.

Over the years, we drew on the strength we found back then to help us navigate living in partnership and raising a family, but never more than when sepsis nearly took my life.

Faith

Thursday evening, September 20 (4th day in ICU) - Facebook update from Scott:

> Scott: After dialysis, Chris, a pastor friend came by and we made a prayer circle around Katy and prayed over her. They had reduced her sedation and after the prayer she opened her eyes! I said, "Hello! Do you know who this is?" And she nodded "yes"! Was beautiful!!

As I review the family communications from when I was sick, I am continually struck by the many sparks of faith and hope that lit up the darkness. They were helpless to fight the sepsis that was ravaging my body, but they could pray that I would survive. Even as they braced for the worst, my family held space for miracles.

Prayer often arises in my journey, both as a request to the larger community ("Please pray for…") and as a form of self-care. It's a chance to acknowledge and express fears, hopes, anger, and other complex emotions.

Prayer can be a means of connection with oneself, with the community, and with whatever a "higher power" represents to the person praying. Prayer holds a promise that we will never be truly alone or abandoned, no matter how hard things get.

Thursday, September 20 - Scott - text to our daughters:

> Scott: I'm glad to hear you are going to pray. […] It took a significant event (getting sober) to change my perspective on prayer.

> In recovery, you are required to find and embrace a higher power. An energy in the universe greater than yourself. Male or female, human or formless, it doesn't matter so long as you find it.

> This was a difficult step for me in recovery. Where I found God was in the eyes of you and your sister, for whom I have no deeper, purer love. Through your eyes I am brave, strong, honest, and purposeful.

> My experience has been one where a journey with my higher power has given me more peace, clarity, strength, and purpose than a journey alone. I encourage you to experience a spiritual journey, find your higher power. Talk with Her [God]. Give Her your unresolvable problems. Ask Her for strength, courage, patience and clarity. I hope it helps you on your journey.

> Daughter: I am excited to go to [a nearby chapel to pray].... I am hoping it will help me feel less helpless for this whole situation and help me find a purpose and role in mom's healing moving forward. Thank you for texting me that, it means a lot.

This message, written when my life hung in the balance, is a beautiful example of how tragedy can open a space for deeper connection: with each other, with ourselves, and with a higher power.

Spiritual Support

In addition to the prayers dedicated to me and my healing throughout my sepsis recovery, I know of at least one prayer-like ritual at a full moon "goddess gathering" in Spokane, attended by my dear friend Heidi. All the women present put their hands in the center of the circle of women to physically move the energy, envisioning the blood circulating through my body, helping to heal my extremities.

Friends have also mentioned things like sound baths, meditation, and yoga, which helped them focus their energy and facilitate healing visualizations on my behalf. Hearing about all the different ways my community was supporting me on a spiritual level, in addition to all their help in the physical realm, meant the world to me.

Knowing that the people who cared about me hadn't given up hope and that they were praying for me and visualizing a full recovery, bolstered my confidence tremendously. And seeing them reconnect with their spirituality brought meaning to what felt like an otherwise senseless tragedy.

Saturday, September 22 - Scott - text to our daughters:

Scott: Also, find a spot for prayer or meditation in your day. Connect with someone who can help you in calm, quiet reflection, where you can seek help from a higher power. Talk with friends. Reach out to family. Prayer will help you move through this each day. We love you both so much!!

Daughters: This weekend has been a really good retreat for us. We have had so much fun! Dad I saw a doe and two fawns last night! Less than 15 feet away from me. So so cute.

Scott: So amazing! I'm so glad you both are there. Nature is so emotionally nourishing, what a perfect time to feed your souls with natural beauty. So great. Makes me and your mom so happy.

Daughters: Thank you so much, Dad.

When Scott told me about the doe and the two fawns the girls had seen, I was overcome with emotion. It felt like Mother Nature herself was sending my girls a message of hope and love, letting them know that they, like those two fawns, still had their mother looking over them, and always would.

There are countless names for deliberately sending your mental and emotional energy toward a positive outcome. For my family, that word is prayer. Whatever you call it, and whatever your beliefs, where you focus your energy during a recovery process matters – not just for the patient, but for the person asking for help or sending positive energy into the world.

The Magic of Mindset

"Whether you think you can, or you think you can't, you're right."

– Henry Ford

Too often, we limit our abilities to what we think makes sense for us, based on our past experiences. And then we wonder why we can't seem to break out of the patterns that keep us stuck in a rut.

This is especially dangerous during the healing process. Placing mental limitations on our potential for recovery, or taking on a projected prognosis as an inevitable outcome, can lead to self-fulfilling prophecies. That's one of the reasons my family worked so hard to shield me from what often seemed like impossible odds, allowing me to hang on to hope for as long as possible.

Picturing a Positive Outcome

Visualizing a full recovery isn't just important for the person recovering, but for everyone involved in their care. Seeing me in the ICU looking so swollen and sick made my daughters concerned that the hospital staff only knew me as this frail, critically ill version of myself. To help them envision me fully recovered, the girls ordered 8 x 10" prints of the most vibrant photos of me they could find. Action shots of me paddle-boarding and bike riding, along with family photos of recent high school and college graduations, framed the whiteboard listing my medical diagnoses and pending procedures. They wanted everyone who interacted with me to see me as a healthy mother with a loving family, not just the deathly ill patient whose life they were trying to save.

Dani and Jordan hung those photos not just for the medical team to see how healthy I had been and could be again, but also so everyone could be reminded to lift me up in prayer and visualize me healthy again. People who entered the room commented on the photos and how nice it was to see what I looked like when I was healthy. They asked the girls where the images were taken and learned about our family. It helped them get to know all of us better and strengthened our connection.

An all-too-common occurrence in medicine is for clinicians struggling with burnout to dehumanize their patients, referring to them as "the pneumonia in bed one" or "the DIC in bed two." Before you become too critical of this, ask yourself if maybe you've done the same by referring to a doctor as "the grumpy lady," or "the old guy with glasses." Medical personnel are human too.

My daughters' simple act helped the hard-working staff and visitors to pause, take in those images of my past successes, and imagine my future potential. It allowed all those who came into contact with me to see beyond my diagnosis. When they looked at the pictures, they saw gratitude, love, and most importantly, hope.

Respect the Process

Tuesday, September 25 - Facebook update from Scott:

> When rested, Katy is lucid, engaged and determined. When fatigued she becomes frail and often confused. She was so tired today that when asked how her lungs felt by the doctor, she looked at me and barely audibly answered, "I forgot my phone...." / Emotionally, her mind is trying to process the incomprehensible horror of the past, present and future that this experience will put her through. With Katy's strength, positivity and support, I have no doubt she will get through this, but undoubtedly her emotional recovery is certain to be a long road. Please pray for courage, peace and acceptance for Katy on her difficult undertaking of emotional mending.

As I became increasingly aware of my situation, under Maren's advisement, Scott and Dani made it clear to everyone who visited that I was to lead all discussions about my medical status and recovery. No one was to bring up possible results with me. This would allow me to focus on my healing without worrying about the future, which was still unknown. They didn't need to worry about me asking, though, because I was too afraid to face anything beyond getting through each day.

As a natural optimist, I was initially hopeful for a full recovery. And for good reason: within a week of waking up at Queen's, my kidneys and lungs were functioning fully despite the damage to them from the septic shock and DIC. This minor miracle bolstered my hopes that, despite the dire appearance of my feet and hands, they could still be saved.

See You Later, ICU

Wednesday, September 26 - Facebook update from Jordan:

> GOOD NEWS!!! Mom is out of the ICU and into her new room in the hospital. She still has a long way to go, but we can finally start sending her flowers.

To say that I received some flowers after posting this on Facebook would be an enormous understatement. The first group of flowers was delivered to my room by five volunteers, each holding two vases. The flowers filled nearly every surface in the space.

And to my surprise, a huge gift box from Nordstrom arrived, containing the softest blanket I had ever felt. The powder-pink blanket, made by Barefoot Dreams, was accompanied by a note from Marnie, Julia, and their family. They had chosen this blanket because Julia had received one just like it while she was in the hospital after her sepsis battle, and it had comforted her throughout her entire journey. They wished the same for me.

The colorful flowers and comforting blanket served as symbols of the new life I was beginning outside of the ICU, and helped me access some of my lost joy as we celebrated my survival. Leaving the ICU signaled the end of my acute medical emergency and the beginning of my long road to recovery. But those gifts made one thing abundantly clear: I would not be traveling that road alone.

September 26 - Facebook update from Scott:

> Katy is having short-term memory issues today. Likely a combo of no sleep, physical trauma, emotional trauma, meds and ICU delirium. Likelihood is everything gets better as she gets out of the ICU circus, off meds and better rested. But she's scared. Holly is doing a superhuman job of calming her and talking with her. Truly incredible watching Holly's calm, powerful strength. So thankful for her.

Even though I was on the road to recovery, I was far from out of the woods.

Scott heard so many medical professionals use this phrase that he finally asked one of the doctors what it meant to be "in the woods."

The doctor replied frankly, "It means she could die at any moment."

Now that I was settled into my new room, Holly said her goodbyes and returned home, filled with hope. She was replaced by three of my favorite people: my dad, my nephew Darrick, and Dani, who returned from California to join Scott as one of my primary advocates.

I wanted to be strong for my family because I knew how scary it must be for them to see me so sick. I wanted them to reassure my mom and Jordan, who couldn't be with me, that I would be okay.

I tried to be strong, but honestly, I wasn't; I didn't feel well at all. I was struggling with my role in the family, feeling like I should take care of them when I needed them to take care of me. My complicated feelings were made worse by the lingering ICU delirium, not to mention the ongoing physical crises wreaking havoc on my organs.

One Organ at a Time

Now that my blood oxygen levels were under control, my focus shifted to my kidneys. A few years prior, I had lost a friend to kidney failure, so the possibility of that happening to me felt real. I was terrified of ending up on dialysis for the rest of my life, or worse, dying as my friend had.

My doctors would come every morning to check on me and update my family with the latest test results. I didn't understand a lot of what was being discussed, but I became obsessed with my kidney function. I worried compulsively about it, day and night.

I was on intermittent kidney dialysis and had to be taken down to the kidney center to be connected to the dialysis equipment for up to four hours each day. Initially, I could only lie down for the process due to my weakness, but over time, I was gradually able to sit up. I remember feeling claustrophobic as I was connected to a piece of equipment that filtered excess fluid and waste from my blood. It worked outside of my body like an artificial kidney.

Each morning, I was so anxious to hear whether my kidneys were regaining strength that I would wake up early in anticipation of my kidney doctor's arrival. The nephrologist was petite and wore tiny ballet flats, so I could see her feet beneath the curtain at my entry door as she quietly shuffled into my room at the crack of dawn each day. She was almost always the first doctor to visit. And each morning, I was pleased to hear that my kidney function was improving.

Wasting Away

I had become obstinate about not wanting to eat because I felt nauseated from the antibiotics and medications, and because the food on my kidney-safe diet was bland and unappealing. Scott and Holly had been trying to feed me, but the food was making me throw up, so I eventually quit eating solid food altogether and would only sip soups and protein drinks.

Because the resulting malnutrition was interfering with my recovery, Scott assigned my nephew Darrick the thankless job of trying to get me to eat, figuring I was less likely to get mad at him for it. I thought of Darrick and Dad as my guests, just like Maren and Holly, so I was trying to be on my best behavior with them. Darrick and my dad were also elected to brush my ratty, matted hair because I was already angry at Scott for "pulling my hair" earlier, and they wanted to keep Dani on my good side so that she could continue to provide me with nurturing emotional support.

Despite Darrick's best efforts at turning eating into a game, I continued to avoid it and to vomit up much of what I did eat. He did make some headway with my hair, though, and everyone agreed I was nicer to him and my dad than I had been to Scott when he tried to detangle it.

Fighting for a Miracle

Facebook update from Scott:

> A big event for Katy is her first session in the Hyperbaric Tank. This procedure puts her in a pressurized vault (looks like a [small] airplane cockpit and she watches TV) that will increase her blood-oxygen levels 5x normal atmospheric pressure. This procedure hopes to increase O2 blood levels in her hands and feet and help Katy's body heal the damaged tissue there. She had to be listed as "stable" to use the Hyperbaric, which she achieved this morning. So a big day for Katy. She is sleeping calmly as I write this. Please lift up this beautiful person in your prayers. Love to you all.

For the first three weeks at Queen's, I endured excruciating treatments in an attempt to save my hands and feet. Nitroglycerin cream[1] was applied to my extremities every eight hours, starting while I was

1. Nitroglycerin is a vasodilator that can open blood vessels, potentially increasing oxygen delivery. It has been used off-label as a cream applied to the skin of tissue that has been damaged by loss of blood flow in an attempt to increase oxygen delivery. It was considered a salvage therapy for me - a sort of "Hail Mary" that could possibly heal tissue that hadn't responded to primary treatments.

in the ICU. It made my hands and feet burn and left me dizzy as the chemicals seeped through my skin. The cream needed to remain on my hands for 45 minutes, an unbearably long time. Over time, these treatments became even more painful as the skin on my hands and feet began to peel away.

Meanwhile, now that I was out of the ICU, hyperbaric oxygen therapy treatments[2] could begin, which we were hopeful could help heal the damage in my lungs and other organs, as well as my hands and feet.

But when Scott asked when I was scheduled for my first hyperbaric treatment, he was told my insurance had declined hyperbaric oxygen therapy for me.

"How much are the treatments?" Scott asked, reaching for his wallet. "I'll put it on my credit card."

"I'm afraid it doesn't work like that," he was told. "We aren't authorized to begin the treatments until they've been approved."

Undeterred, Scott escalated the conversation to the head intensivist in charge of my treatment program, who ultimately agreed to go ahead and start the treatments immediately, regardless of whether or not they would eventually be reimbursed.

I often wonder about patients who don't have this kind of unrelenting advocacy on their side. What happens to them when their insurance company decides their hospital can't perform the life-and-limb-saving procedures they need?

After many days of these challenging treatments, my hands started to reveal a healthy pink color where the skin had peeled away. The purple started to fade on my palms, the backs of my hands, and even the base of my fingers. The remaining damaged tissue on my hands

---

2. Hyperbaric oxygen chambers deliver pure oxygen at an increased atmospheric pressure, administering higher oxygen levels to the blood and tissues, which promotes the healing of a variety of conditions.

was in the blackened fingertips, which I already knew I would lose. But my hands, including both of my thumbs, had been saved!

My spirits were further bolstered by news from my nephrologist and pulmonologist that my kidneys and lungs were functioning normally. No more dialysis!

Unfortunately, the news was not so good for my feet. Although I wasn't able to see my feet as well as I could see my hands, I knew my toes were dry and blackish-purple like my fingertips, and my feet were still grotesquely pointed away from my body.

I learned that my feet had a different type of damage than my hands, called wet gangrene, which was far more dangerous than the dry gangrene on my fingertips. I started to get large, open sores on the magenta flesh on top of my feet, and my medical team was concerned that it could lead to sepsis again. They were on high alert, checking on me regularly for even the most minor signs of infection. We wanted to try to save my feet, but not at the risk of losing my life, which was a possibility because my body was so depleted.

Slowly, the reality began to seep in that, despite all our efforts and prayers, my feet might not come back to life as my hands had. From the first day I woke up in the ICU, I had heard my doctors say that the soles of my feet were black, but I had locked that horrifying information into a vault in my brain. I couldn't handle it. Not yet, anyway.

Hope, faith, prayer, and community support gave me the strength to dig deep within myself, finding the grit I needed to keep moving forward despite the darkness in my soles, my hands, and my life.

Photos

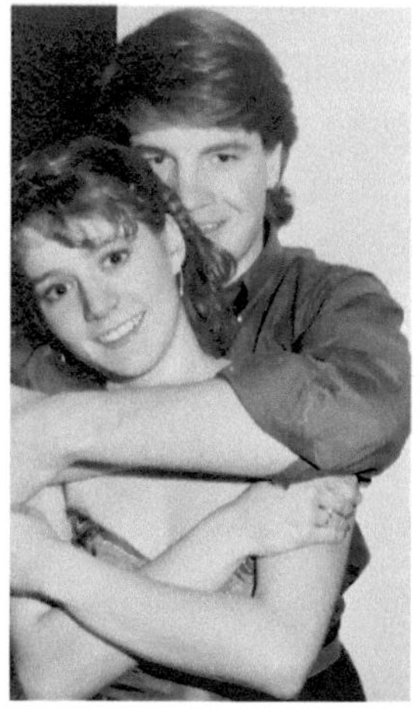

Katy and Scott - College dance, 1985

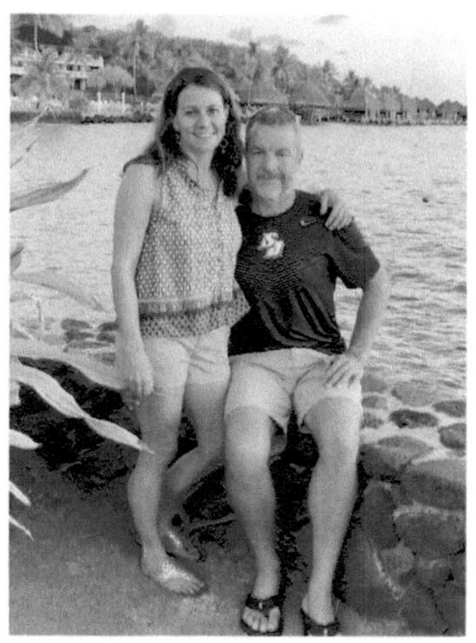

Katy and Scott - Tahiti, one month before sepsis, August 2018

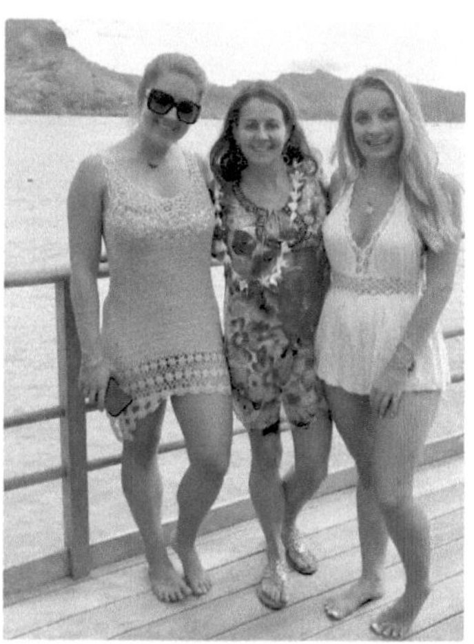

Dani, Katy, and Jordan - Tahiti, August 2018

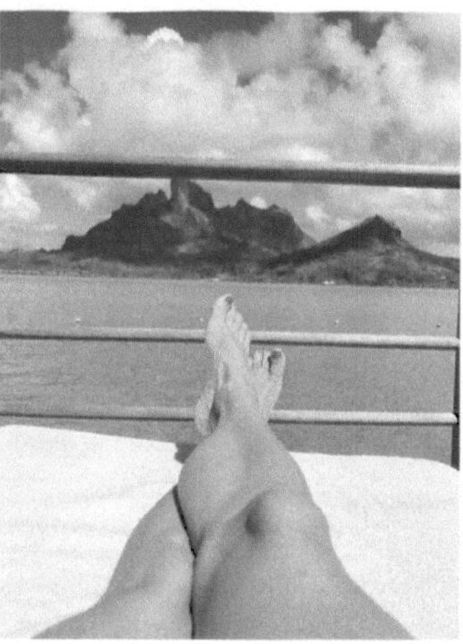

Katy's legs - Tahiti, August 2018

Additional photos at **www.katygrainger.com/book**

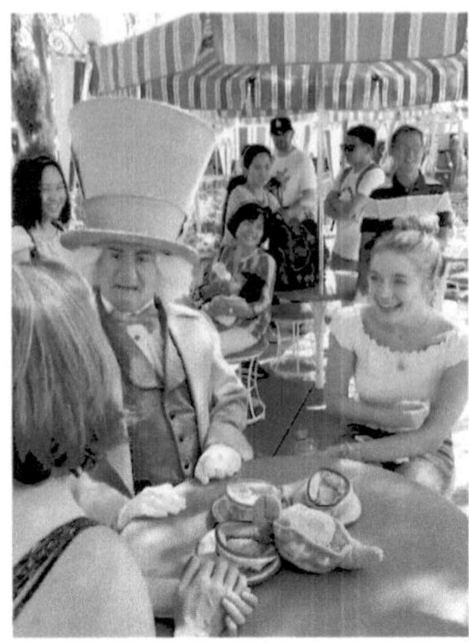

Jordan and The Mad Hatter, Disneyland - Five days before sepsis

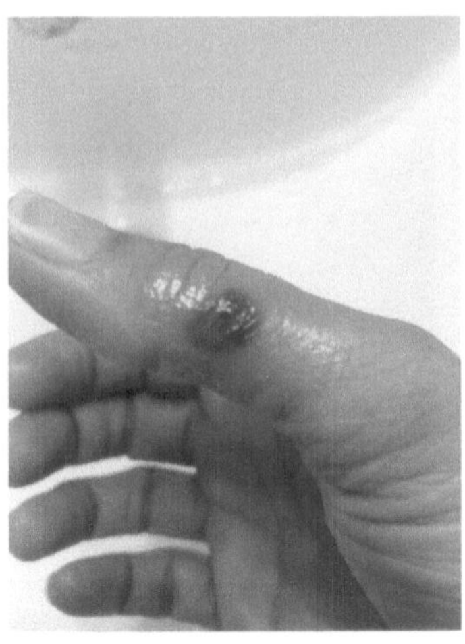

Katy's fingers with the oozing and unusual bump - Friday, September 14, 2018

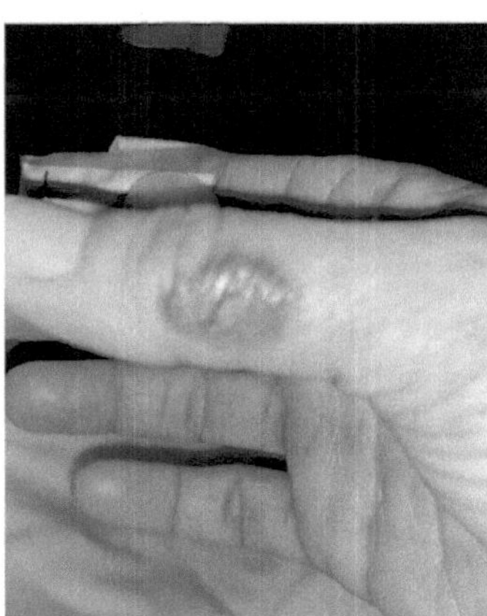

Katy's thumb at Hospital, Kauai - Sunday, September 16

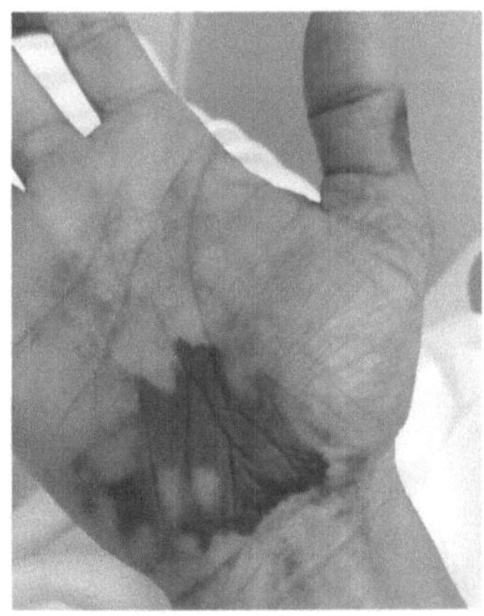

Katy's hand, DIC - Before airlift to Oahu - Monday, September 17

Additional photos at **www.katygrainger.com/book**

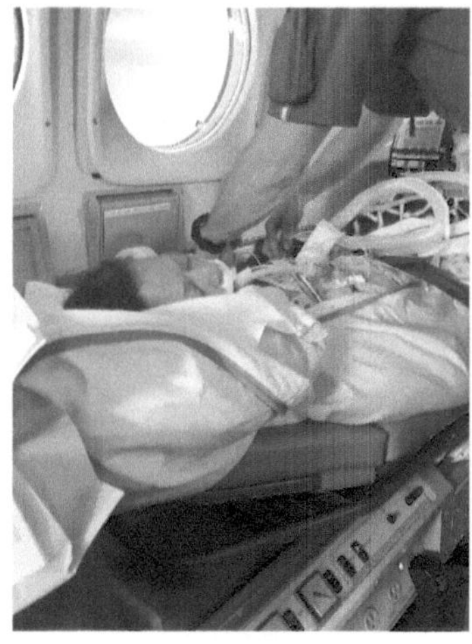

Katy intubated in medically induced coma - Transport to ICU on Oahu

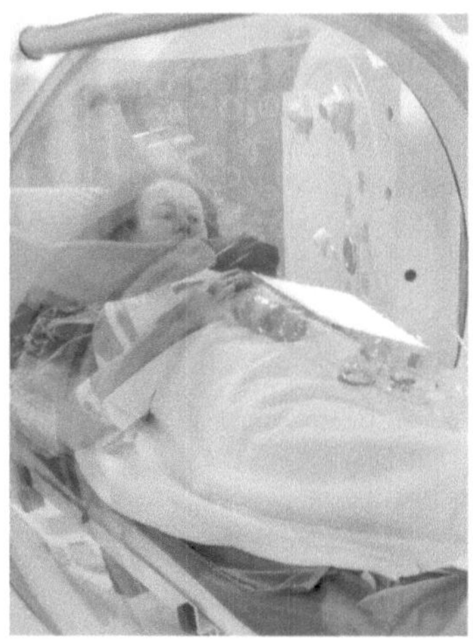

Post ICU - Katy in hyperbaric chamber, Queen's Medical Center

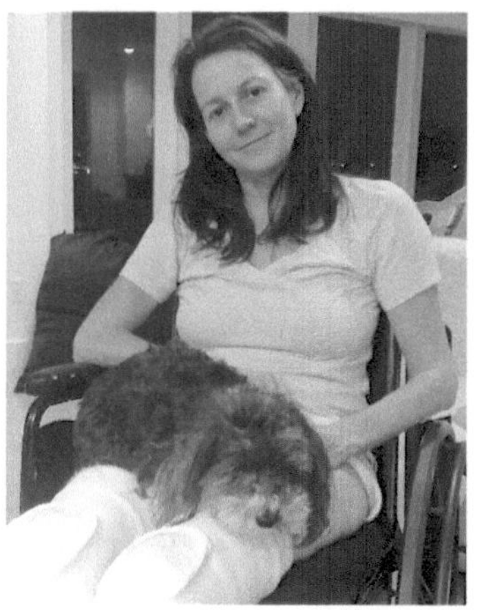

Home with Cody comforting me - November 2018

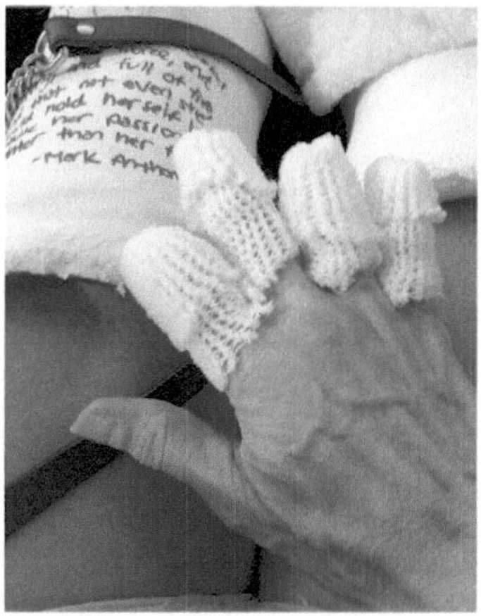

Fingers were amputated one month after leg amputations - November 2018

Additional photos at **www.katygrainger.com/book**

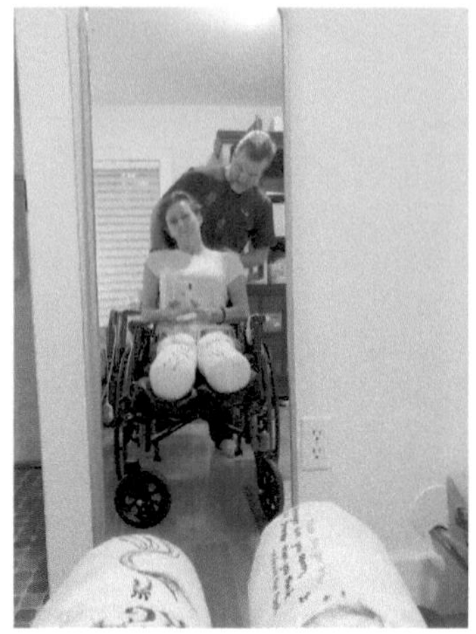

Scott brushing my hair after finger amputations - December 2018

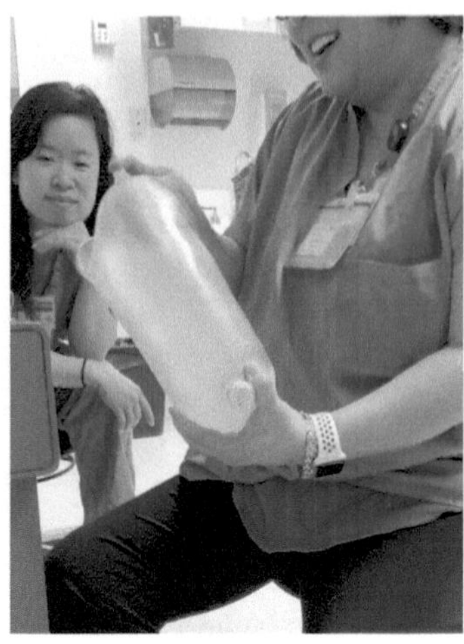

My prosthetist fitting my first legs - December 27, 2018

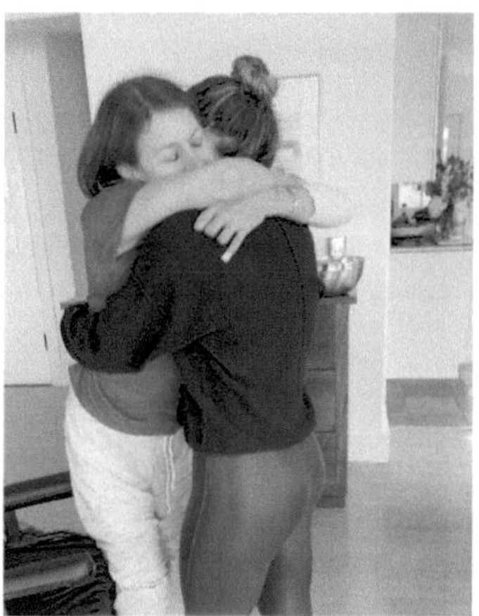

Standing with Jordan on my new legs - December 27, 2018

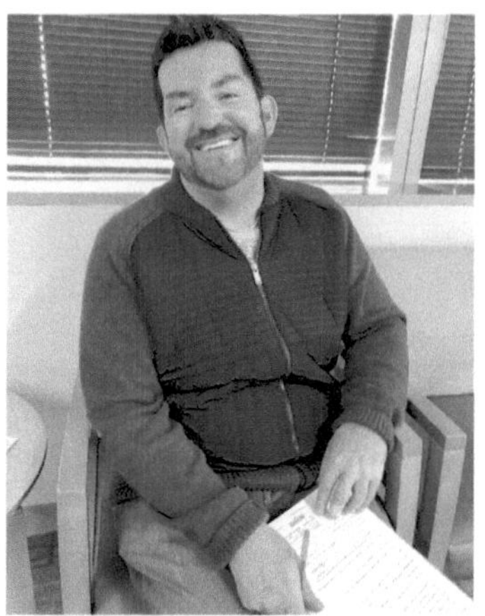

Nurse Todd at one of a million appointments - 2018

Additional photos at **www.katygrainger.com/book**

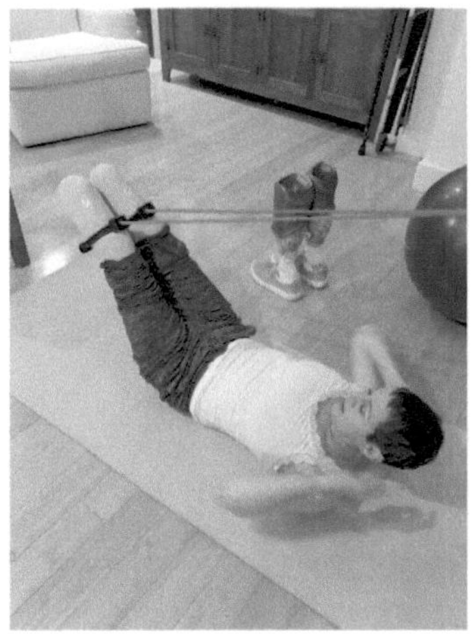

Strengthening my body with my new short hair - 2019

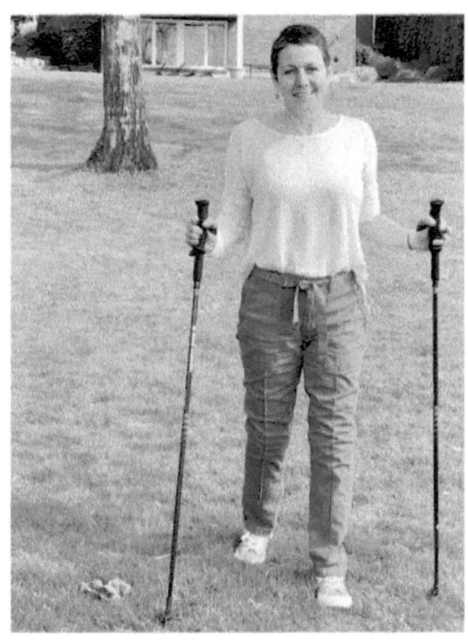

Walking with walking sticks - March 2019

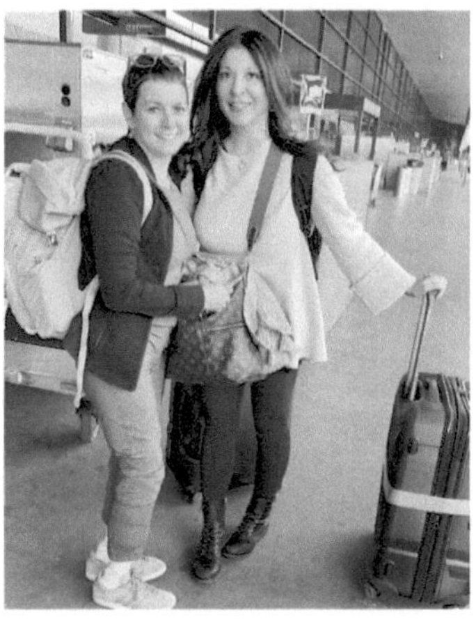

Midori and Katy, ready to fly to Rome - Three months after first prosthetic legs, April 2019

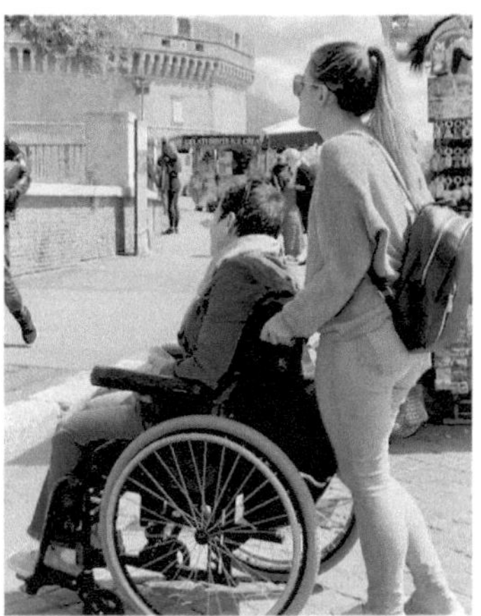

Katy and Jordan - Rome, April 2019

Additional photos at **www.katygrainger.com/book**

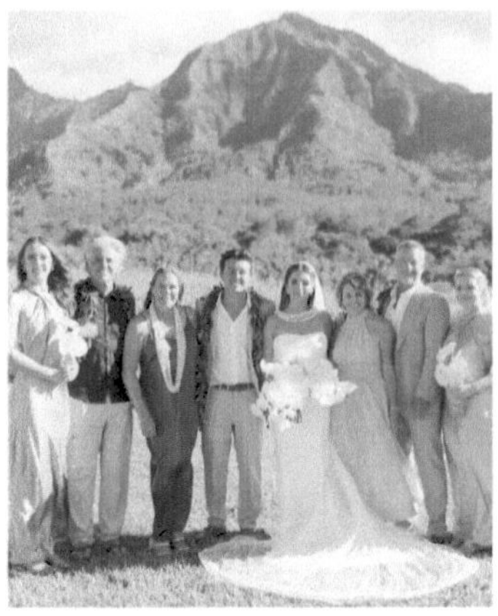

Dani and Hunter's wedding - Hanalei, HI, June 2022

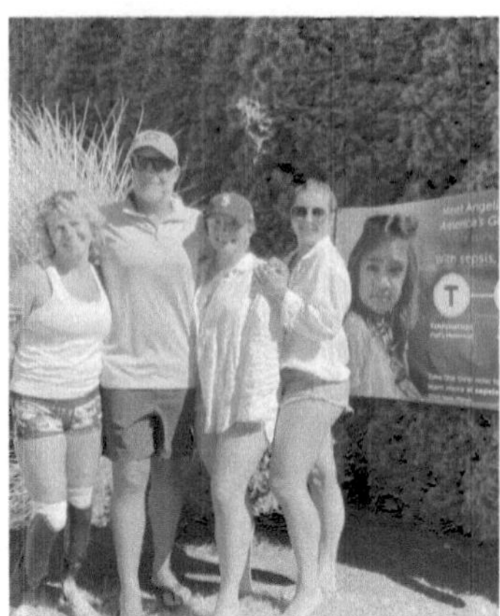

Family Sepsis Superheroes Fundraiser

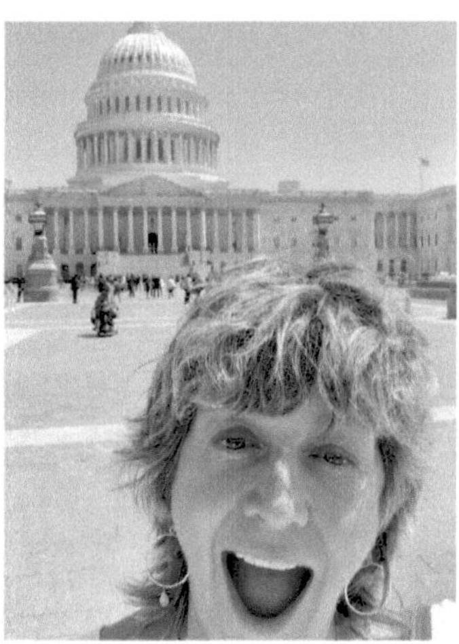

Lobbying for Sepsis Alliance in Washington, DC

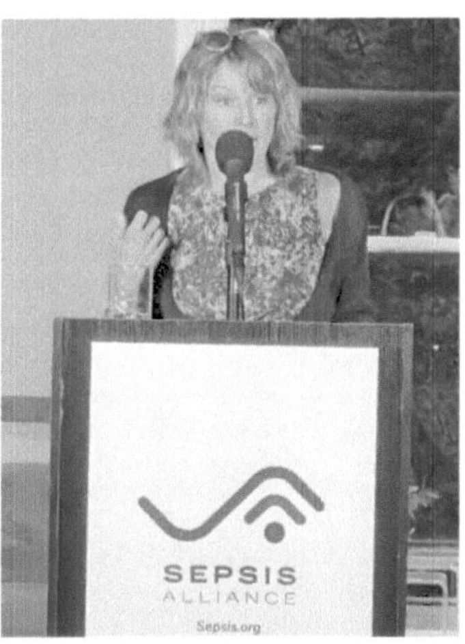

Speaking in Washington DC for sepsis advocacy awareness

Additional photos at **www.katygrainger.com/book**

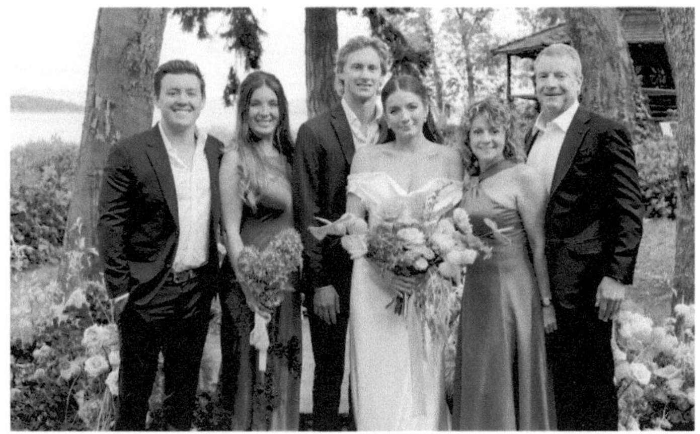

Jordan and Kai's Wedding - Whidbey Island, WA, October 2024

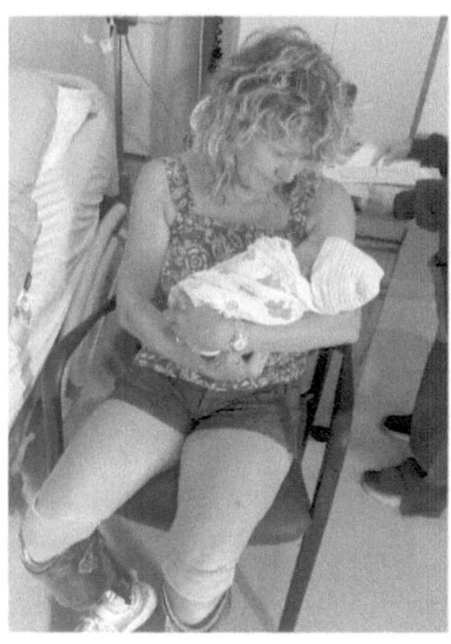

My dream: holding my first grandchild on his birthday - March 2025

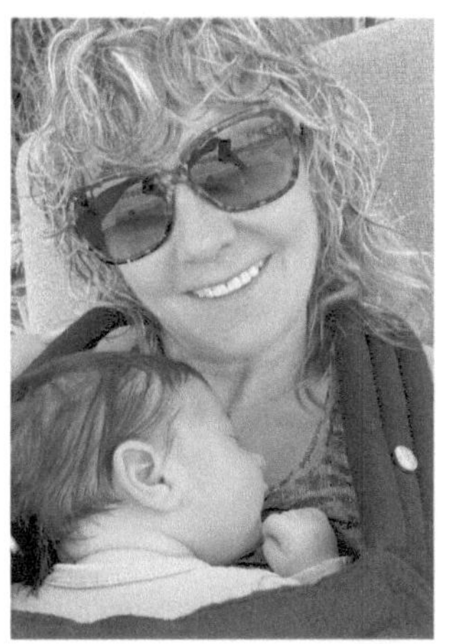

Grateful for every day of my life. I wouldn't be where I am today if all this hadn't happened!

Additional photos at **www.katygrainger.com**

CHAPTER 12

UNDEFEATED

"You will face many defeats in life, but never let yourself be defeated."

– Maya Angelou

Endurance

September 24 - Scott and Marnie text:

Marnie: One doctor gave us advice I go back to whenever we ask the "what ifs": you can't go back. You can only go forward and live life to its fullest. It's overwhelming now, but you'll get to the other side of this and rise up from there.

Scott: So true. No other way but forward. And HOW we do it is up to us.

Marnie: And I know you guys. You will do it with great attitudes (and maybe a tiny bit of wallowing because sometimes you can't avoid it), but you will move onward and upward!

Grit and resilience come down to endurance. Healing is a marathon, not a sprint. It's a long road to recovery. We have to pace ourselves so we don't burn out.

There will be times when we just have to keep going, even though we feel like we have nothing left to give. These are the moments when we start to think: *That's it, I don't have the strength. I can't do this.* That's our opportunity to find our grit.

We have to keep moving forward, even if it's just one tiny step at a time, trusting the rest will come.

Challenging Denial

September 24 - Maren - text to Scott:

Maren: Has she started to realize how bad her hands and feet are?

Scott: Yes that is setting in. She has taken her gloves off several times today and stares at them.

Maren: Oh my heart breaks for her. And for you and for all of us. Wish I could be there to support you both. I love you so much! And I'm so impressed with your strength.
Hers too!

I remember one day in the hospital when a young nurse came into my room and placed a device on my ankle that allowed us to hear the repeating thump-swoosh of my blood flowing toward my feet. The first time we'd gone through this routine reminded me of the first time we had heard our daughters' heartbeats when they were each the size of a bean inside my body. It was a sound of hope and promise.

But then, as he slowly moved the microphone down my calf, past the bright pink skin of my ankle and onto the deep purple skin on the top of my foot, the heartbeat sound stopped dead. A terrible silence fell over the room.

The vault in my brain where I had been storing all my doubts came flying open. I knew what it meant, that deafening silence. But it was too painful to admit it, to feel the excruciating disappointment and hopelessness, so I tried to stuff all the heartbreak back into that vault.

But how could I ignore it when that awful experience was repeated daily?

On this particular day, I snapped at the young nurse, saying, "Can you just stop doing that?! Can you quit coming in here?! It's not going to make any sound! I don't want to hear that anymore!"

His eyes widened, and he nodded as he pulled the device away from my foot. When he quickly turned away from me, I saw his eyes begin to well up with tears as he rushed out of my room. I knew I had hurt his feelings and felt horrible for talking to him that way. But my world had just been shattered. I could no longer keep it in.

In trying to ease my pain, I had lashed out at him and then retreated back to the safety of denial. I wasn't ready to give up hope. I was protecting myself from a truth I wasn't prepared to accept. Our minds have amazing ways of shielding us from the things we aren't ready to handle.

Looking back now, I realize my nurse had just witnessed the heart-wrenching moment when I finally confronted the reality that my feet couldn't be saved. His tears were for me, not for him.

Betting It All on a Longshot

September 28 - Facebook update from Scott:

> We are strictly focused on doing the daily work. That's it. Not future tripping about "what happens if..." Just doing the work.

Even so, the emotional trauma of what happened and an unclear future is often overwhelming. I would in two seconds, and wish I could, trade places with her. And I believe that those who love her really don't care whatsoever what future setbacks she may have.

She will always be Katy. But the magnitude of the whole thing sometimes overwhelms her. So hard to see.

Each morning, I reviewed my daily schedule on the whiteboard in my room, praying I would be scheduled for a hyperbaric treatment. We were holding out hope that hyperbarics could heal my feet. I went as often as they could get me into one of the two lie-flat chambers, which allowed me to stay on a gurney since I was too weak to sit up. They didn't have room for me every day, but most days they were able to fit me in.

At the scheduled time, a patient transport worker would transfer me from my bed to a gurney and take me to the hyperbaric chambers, which seemed to be about a mile away from my room. We went down elevators, through long hallways, and left the main hospital building to cross the lovely, park-like setting of the Queen's Medical Center campus. The contrast of the sterile hospital with the beautiful outdoors of Hawaii made my heart ache for the life I had before sepsis. I prayed my treatments would work and I would be able to live a full life, spending time in nature again.

I was greeted by the same technician every day. He was aware of my situation and treated me with tender loving care. Because the equipment was so sensitive and needed to remain sterilized, he helped me change out of my hospital gown before every treatment. He carefully traded my old gown for a new one wrapped in sterile packaging, being careful not to expose my emaciated naked body underneath. He removed the socks covering my purple feet and hands and replaced the rubber band that held my hair out of my face with one he'd made for me out of a sterilized elastic bandage. I was unable to help because of my damaged hands and feet, but the routine didn't seem to bother him at all.

We talked about family and life in Hanalei, and shared stories about The Queen's Medical Center. He had worked on my hospital floor, so he asked after the nurses, reassuring me that they were all dedicated to the patients they served. He also told me stories about working with other patients like me, which made me feel less alone in my extreme situation.

What we didn't talk about were my condition, my progress, or my odds of making a full recovery. I couldn't bear to imagine a world where these treatments didn't work for me.

Regaining my Wits

Monday, October 1 - Facebook update from Scott:

> Yesterday marked two complete weeks since the morning Tiffany found Katy in a semi-conscious state in Hanalei and drove her to Wilcox Hospital....
>
> The big news over the weekend pertains to Katy's mental and emotional improvement. As of Sunday she has no symptoms of ICU Delirium and is back with us as the Katy we all love so much.
>
> Her hallucinations, paranoia, anxiety, and insomnia are no longer tormenting her, and she has regained much of the sparkle and warm energy that defines her, even in the extremely difficult confines of her condition. It's wonderful to have her back.

It was a relief for me, my family, and my medical team when I finally began to think clearly again. We could now count my brain among the organs that had recovered from the damage caused by the sepsis and DIC. I was relieved to put the confusion and paranoia behind me, and we were all delighted that my dad got to see me back to my old self before he returned to the mainland. My mom was so worried and would be thrilled to learn that, despite the damage to my fingers and feet, I was still me.

Dad and Darrick left after the weekend, but not before my friend Laurie arrived from the Big Island to help us for the week. Laurie is Hunter's mom; she and I met six years earlier when our kids began dating, and we've been close friends ever since.

I was continually surprised by the never-ending parade of my favorite people coming to see me every few days. Now that I was thinking more clearly, I was able to fully appreciate the gift of their time and the care they gave to my family and me.

When I look back at my stay in the hospital and recovery, my visitors are what I remember most. They bolstered my mental health, helped me with my physical needs, distracted me from my despair, and reassured me they would be with me through my recovery, regardless of the outcome.

The Most Painful Words I've Ever Said

I remember my final day taking that gurney ride to the hyperbaric chamber. Sometimes I went alone, but that day, Scott was by my side. Maybe he knew. I don't know how because we didn't talk about it, but he seemed to understand my mind better than I did since my hospitalization.

I remember being brought into the room on my gurney and exchanging all my clothes and equipment for sterilized versions of the same items as usual. I was trying to work up the courage to say what I needed to say, but I knew that once I admitted it, I could never take it back. As they placed the heated blanket over me, I tried to muster the strength, but I couldn't say the words.

They transferred me to the special gurney that goes inside the hyperbaric chamber, and I felt my last chance slipping away. Without thinking about it, I reached out and grabbed Scott's arm as I sobbed, "I don't want to do this anymore. I don't want to go in there."

He looked at me, stunned. I saw the recognition and grief in his eyes as I blurted out the hardest words I have ever had to say:

"I know we can't save my feet."

Time stopped as my words hung in the air.

Scott looked at me with his beautiful blue eyes brimming with tears. He put his forehead against mine and said, "It's okay, Babe, you don't need to do this anymore. I love you. Everything is going to be okay."

He thanked my friend for taking such good care of me and declared, "We're done here today. We're going back to our room." They transferred me back onto the other gurney and let me return to my room with my new sterilized gown and socks, with Scott by my side.

I felt hopeless, staring ahead in a daze as stark hallways and unfamiliar people passed by my gurney. We left the sterile light of the air-conditioned building and passed beneath the robin's egg blue sky and green tree canopy of the Queen's campus. The echoing of the halls was replaced with the hopeful sound of birdsong.

It was impossible to ignore the contrast of my hospital world with the world I longed to reenter. The sun-drenched outdoors seemed to mock the darkness of my situation as we entered the main hospital building and returned to my room.

I was transferred to the safety of my bed and tucked into my plush blankets, surrounded by cards and flowers, and photos of Scott, Dani, Jordan, and me in happier times. Thanks to Dani's thoughtful touches in my room, I breathed in the scent of lavender essential oil and heard soft music playing on my new portable speaker. I took a few calming breaths and allowed my mind to return to the present.

Very cautiously, Scott began to talk to me about our future. He knew how sad and out of control I felt, and wanted to let me know he'd been quietly preparing for the long road to recovery ahead. He invited my input, gently reassuring me that I would be the one to choose our next steps.

I was overcome with gratitude as it became clear to me how long he'd been anticipating this conversation, and how patiently he had waited for me to be ready to have it with him.

I love Scott, my family, and my medical team so much for protecting my heart and letting me accept my recovery at my own pace. It was so compassionate of them to give me the time I needed to try to save my feet and to allow me to realize on my own when it was time to stop treatment. I know they all held out hope with me, and I will forever be grateful for the time I was given to come to terms with what was happening to my body.

The Next Step

Now that I had begun to accept the reality that I would lose my feet and the blackened portions of my fingers, it was time to look at our options. We wouldn't use the word amputations until much later. I wasn't ready, and my team was waiting for me to introduce this charged word into our discussions. So, Scott simply asked me, "Where would you like to have your surgeries?"

He presented the three most sensible options: remaining on Oahu, returning to Kauai, or moving back to Seattle.

With broken hearts, we ruled out the idea of returning to Kauai. It was such a small island, and the surgeons there weren't likely to have had a lot of experience with this type of surgery. Based on Scott's research, there also didn't appear to be anyone on the island who made prosthetic limbs. Besides, our home was an hour from the hospital, so getting me the care and support I needed would be an ongoing logistical nightmare.

It also didn't make sense to stay in Honolulu or anywhere else on Oahu. Despite the first-rate medical care we were receiving, we didn't have friends and family there, or a home where my family could live and where I could recover. Our friends would soon need back the condo we'd been borrowing. We were grateful for the use of this beautiful home while I recovered, but it was never intended to be a long-term solution.

That left us with the option of returning to Seattle, which had a highly respected regional trauma center more than capable of performing my amputations and taking care of my rehabilitation and prosthetic needs. We would also be closer to our extended family. Scott discussed the decision with me, allowing me to reach the inevitable conclusion on my own.

"Returning to Seattle does make a lot of sense, but isn't Midori living in our house?"

When we'd first left for Hawaii, we'd thought of it as a temporary adventure away from home, so we rented the house to friends, leaving the door open for our eventual return. But as the years stretched on and more and more friends cycled through, it became clear that "home" had shifted in our minds, and that we weren't all that keen on being landlords. When our most recent tenant left unexpectedly in August, Midori floated the idea of selling her much larger home and buying ours. Now that her boys were grown and gone, she could downsize and retire, and we would always have a place to stay when we were in town. It was a win-win situation.

"Don't worry," he reassured me, "we've got it all figured out."

"Really?"

"It was all Midori's idea," he said with a big smile. "We were at the condo talking about the future while you were in the ICU, and she said, 'You need to move back to Seattle. I'm moving out of your house, and you're moving back in. It's the perfect solution. It's meant to be. My house was on the market for a month, and I didn't even get a nibble. The universe has spoken. You need to move back to be close to family and your kids while Katy recovers.' And the best part is," he went on, his voice breaking a little, "she promised not to sell her house for two years so that she can be next door to help us as long as we need her."

That commitment floored me. Not only would she need to move her things back to her house, but she would also need to delay her retirement. And she was agreeing to care for me for two years on top of everything else?! I couldn't believe all that she had done and was willing to do for our family.

Still, obstacles kept plaguing my weary mind. "But what about the sunken patio between the garage and the house?" I couldn't imagine crossing that rift in a wheelchair.

Scott pulled out his phone and showed me a picture of a brand-new walkway that had been erected in anticipation of my arrival, creating a smooth path directly from the garage to the kitchen door.

"But there's no shower on the main floor," I fretted.

Scott assured me he had already thought of that too, explaining that my brother-in-law, Dan, was coming up to Seattle from Salem to install a portable shower he had found online, specially designed for a wheelchair.

"I'll need a hospital bed…"

Once again, Scott was one step ahead of my anxieties. Dani had already arranged for a hospital bed and rolling table, just like the ones in my hospital room, to be brought to our Mercer Island house if I decided to go there.

It was clear to me that a lot of thought had gone into their preparations and that the Seattle area made the most sense for my recovery. I could tell that, although they would respect whatever decision I made, Scott and the girls had done their homework and long since agreed that returning to Mercer Island was the best option for all of us.

I was comforted by the prospect of being surrounded by my family and old friends. It was hard being in Hawaii when I knew my parents and other family members were thousands of miles away back in Washington state. After 10 years away, I had begun to believe that

Seattle was no longer our home, but now it was clear that my deepest roots were there.

As sad as I was to leave Hawaii, I knew what the answer had to be.

"If Midori's really willing to move back to her house, and to help us, let's go back to Seattle."

"Done," Scott said with a gentle smile.

And so it was.

Going Back to Get Ahead

Healing is not the neat, linear process we think it should be. It's chaotic, and often loops back on itself. Sometimes moving forward looks like moving backward, and sometimes getting where we're going means having to retrace our steps. Moving back to Seattle was not on my Bingo card, but it turned out to be the step backward I needed to find my way forward.

Likewise, grit doesn't always look the way you think it's going to. Sometimes it looks like digging in and slogging through a painful process, and sometimes it looks like having the courage to finally let go of what isn't working and move forward in a new direction.

CHAPTER 13

A HUI HOU, HAWAII - UNTIL WE MEET AGAIN

"The greatest glory in living lies not in never falling, but in rising every time we fall."

– Nelson Mandela

Seattle Bound

Unbeknownst to me, Marnie had introduced Scott to Dr. Janna Friedly, a doctor at UW Medicine's Rehabilitation Medicine Clinic at Harborview Medical Center in Seattle. They had spoken a few times, discussing our options for surgery and rehabilitation in Seattle. Dr. Friedley had referred us to the top hand and orthopedic surgeons at Harborview, the Level One Trauma Center serving the Northwestern States. Both surgeons performed amputations regularly and were highly regarded in their fields.

When these surgeons agreed to accept me at Harborview and perform my surgeries without seeing me in person beforehand, it was a massive win for our family. Not only would I have world-class doctors, but I would be with my family in the best place to recover from them.

Soon, I would be close to my Seattle friends, Scott's and my extended families, and closer to Jordan and Dani in the familiar home where my girls had grown up before we moved to Hawaii. Washington had been my home for most of my life and was welcoming us back with open arms.

Bureaucracy Blues

One significant obstacle still stood in our way: insurance coverage for my airlift to Seattle. Because The Queen's Medical Center was qualified to perform amputations – "my surgeries," as I still preferred to call them – my health insurance would not cover an air ambulance to transport me from Honolulu to Seattle. They were only willing to cover my transport to Seattle on a commercial airline in a standard seat, with a nurse accompanying me.

At that point, I was still unable to sit upright because of extreme weakness from the lingering effects of sepsis, malnutrition, and a massive bed sore across my bottom, which was still an open wound and a constant concern for infection. Meanwhile, chronic diarrhea ravaged my body because of the strong antibiotics, and there was no way for me to get to a bathroom quickly because of my damaged feet.

Yet my insurance carrier thought transporting me through the airport in a wheelchair, and lifting me into a seat that would be unable to recline as far as I needed, would work just fine. We couldn't imagine any way I'd be able to safely fly to Seattle on a regular flight in my current condition, and the need for surgery was becoming urgent because of the risk of infection in my feet.

No matter how much Scott and my medical team petitioned our insurance company, they would not approve our transport. They preferred to pay for me to have my surgeries in Honolulu and go into a recovery center until I was ready to take a standard plane back to Seattle. The fact that my family and extended support team would have no place to stay in the wildly expensive city of Honolulu while I recovered didn't concern them.

Scott was determined to get me transferred to Harborview safely, one way or another. But it wasn't easy. He faced significant opposition from a system designed to protect the status quo. Because the hospital was waiting on insurance approval, they wouldn't sign my transfer papers. Without transfer papers from Queen's, Harborview in Seattle could not admit me. It was a classic bureaucratic Catch-22, with my life and our finances hanging in the balance.

But Scott didn't give up. He worked with my doctors to choose October 17th as the ideal transfer date. He reached out to an air ambulance company on his own and was told they could transport me as long as both hospitals approved the transfer. To reserve the flight, he would have to pay out of pocket for the plane in advance and in full, with no chance of a refund, since the airplane would be coming from California with medical personnel and would have to return whether I was on it or not. Despite the risk, Scott booked the flight, knowing he had just two days to persuade the administrators at Queen's to sign the transfer paperwork to Harborview despite the lack of insurance approval.

After 36 hours of jumping through bureaucratic hoops, he finally put all the pieces in place for our transfer to Seattle. Meanwhile, I focused on gaining strength for my surgeries, insulated from the precarious state of my transfer. Dr. Friedley was able to talk Harborview into assigning me a bed, with the commitment from Scott that I would be there on the evening of October 17th. Once our hospitalist at Queen's understood that we were paying for the airlift out of pocket, he promised to get the transfer completed.

Scott's aggressive advocacy and initiative paid off, and we were finally given the transfer papers we'd been asking for, along with ambulance transport from Queen's to the air ambulance. I don't fully understand all the magic that went into making my transfer happen, or why it was so hard in the first place, but I know it never would have happened without Scott's tenacity.

We looked into appealing the insurance claim when we returned to Seattle, but were advised against it because our attorney's fees would likely exceed the reimbursement. Ultimately, we realized that focusing on my recovery was more important, so we let it go. After all, accepting what's beyond our control had become a central tenet of our lives.

It breaks my heart that insurance companies can be so insensitive to the suffering of their patients. I count my blessings that we were able to cover an expense that would be unthinkable to so many in my position.

With the flight booked and my transfer papers in hand, we did our best to get some rest, praying that everything would go smoothly and that, the following night, we'd be sleeping in Seattle.

The Transfer

Much to our relief, paramedics arrived in my room at the scheduled time on the morning of October 17 and prepared me for transport. They wrapped me up like a burrito in a red canvas bag designed to protect me from the elements while facilitating smooth transfers between the hospitals and ambulances. *This must be how I arrived from Kauai,* I thought as they wrapped me, glad to be lucid for this transfer.

My transport nurse and paramedics then rushed Scott and me to the airfield via ambulance and loaded me onto the small plane that would fly us to Boeing Field, just south of downtown Seattle. At the same time, Dani and Marnie flew to Seattle on a commercial airline with their suitcases, plus several large duffel bags containing essential belongings from our Hanalei house that Scott had packed on a quick trip to Hanalei.

As our small jet flew above the skyline of Honolulu, I was overcome with overwhelming grief. Honolulu had never been home, but leaving it meant leaving Hawaii, the beloved paradise where my family and I had lived for the past 10 years. Tears blurred my vision. The island of Oahu grew smaller and smaller through my tiny window, as my heart broke for the dreams I was leaving behind.

That was the last thing I remember before awakening six hours later to the familiar sight of the Seattle skyline as we approached.

Welcome Home

The grief I felt leaving Hawaii was soon replaced with the comfort of returning to our prior home with a promise of healing and recovery. When we landed, I was carefully lifted from the tiny airplane into a waiting ambulance as the sun set over the Olympic Mountains to the west. A young paramedic hopped into the ambulance with a huge smile.

"Welcome home, Katy!" she called out.

I smiled back. It felt good to be reminded that I had returned to the city where I had raised my kids and would be close to family and long-time friends.

"I'm a friend of Kirk Robinson," the paramedic went on to explain, "Kirk made me promise to take good care of you. He said to tell you that hundreds of people are praying for you through your church and throughout the Seattle Fire Department."

This message would have been powerful coming from anyone, but the fact that the message was from Kirk especially touched my heart. Kirk was a young man I had met years earlier, when I was a leader on a youth mission trip with him in Mexico. We became friends and kept in touch over the years.

Kirk was dealing with life-threatening health issues of his own. While I was in the hospital, we had been bonding about our personal struggles in text messages and Facebook comments. He had become one of my strongest and most appreciated cheerleaders. I was a big fan of his as well. His welcome message meant the world to me and reassured me that our decision to return to Seattle was the right one.

Harborview

After a 15-minute ambulance ride, I was unloaded onto a gurney and taken to my new room at Harborview Medical Center. My nurse introduced herself and told me she had heard my story from a mutual friend and had been awaiting my arrival. Like Kirk, another old friend of mine had paved the way for our return to Seattle. After many years away, we felt warmly welcomed back into our Seattle community.

As I fell asleep holding Scott's hand, I looked out my window at the buildings of downtown Seattle, watching the familiar spectacle of a Washington State Ferry making its way across the Puget Sound. I could see the building where I worked in my first job out of college, nearly 30 years earlier, as well as the building where my nephew Darrick now worked, since he had moved to Seattle after graduating. I felt comforted knowing I was closer to family and was grateful that Seattle still felt like home.

Being in Seattle meant more than just being home; it meant surgery was imminent. I was going to have to start hearing and using the word I had been avoiding for so long: *amputations*.

My mantra at Harborview became: "The only way out is through."

Meeting My Dream Team

The next morning, my new doctors began visiting me during their rounds. Similar to my experience at Queen's, I had an overwhelming number of people on my care team. Scott had already spoken to several of my doctors while we were still in Hawaii, so plans for my upcoming surgeries were well underway. I was pleased to see the confidence everyone had for me and my situation. I could tell we were in great hands with this team.

Still, I confided in Scott that I was terrified about the surgeries and couldn't imagine losing my feet and my fingertips all at the same time. Despite my brittle fingertips, I was still able to use my hands a little. It seemed like it would be horrible to have them stitched up and in pain while my lower legs were still healing. I didn't feel like I could handle all that at once.

To my great relief, he and my doctors understood my concern and presented me with several options for my surgeries and recovery. I could have all of my surgeries at once, or I could opt to have my hand and foot surgeries done separately. To avoid infection, I would need to have my feet amputated as soon as I was strong enough, but I could decide to wait for a few weeks to do my fingertips because infection was unlikely.

My vocal cords also needed a minor procedure because of damage from being intubated. Like so many things I had taken for granted before this massive wave of loss crashed over my life, struggling to speak made me realize how much I relied on my voice, not just in the practical sense of communicating my needs to those around me, but as a part of my identity. My voice has always been my ambassador in so many ways, and to have it weakened to the point where it could barely be heard made me feel isolated and invisible.

Although I felt empowered to choose what was best for me, these conversations were still tough. Making this decision meant I was agreeing to have parts of my own body removed, a prospect that remained surreal and overwhelming. But I knew I needed to accept what had happened to me and consent to the amputation surgeries so I could move forward in my recovery.

Ultimately, I told Scott I wanted time to fully heal and adjust to one set of missing limbs before moving on to the next, so I chose to do the leg amputations first, then the finger amputations a month later. I also agreed to undergo the procedure on my vocal cords during my leg surgery, hoping that, after a few healing days in silence, my voice would soon become strong again and I might begin feeling more like myself. It felt like a big step forward, having these difficult decisions behind me.

Scott excused himself to schedule my surgery. An hour later, he texted to tell me they wanted to do my leg amputations in just four days. My confidence waned. That felt impossibly soon to me. My mind began looking for excuses to push out the surgery date.

Facing the loss of my lower legs and feet was hard enough, but to do my surgeries when I was still so weak? Was that advisable? Unable to keep much food down, I was still under 90 pounds, despite the efforts of my nutritionist and a whole lot of protein milkshakes, the only thing I could stand to eat.

"Do we have to be solid on this surgery date? Can we push it to the weekend?"

Scott responded immediately, "We're on the right track. Everything is going to be okay."

I knew he was right.

The only way out is through.

Preparing My Body for Surgery

Reassured that my surgery date should be as soon as possible so I could move on with my life, I focused my energy on trying to regain some strength. I had lost significant muscle mass while recovering from the ravages of sepsis, leaving me dangerously thin and frail. My medical team advised me to try to gain back as much of that lost mass as I could before surgery. I had lifted two-pound weights a few times at Queen's, but now, with only a few days until my first surgery, I became more committed to strength training and nutrition.

Most of the time, the idea of food turned my stomach. But every once in a while, I would have a moment of respite from the nausea and realize just how hungry I was. In one of these moments, I heard my nephew Darrick mention to my daughters and my niece that a new burger joint, Seattle's first Shake Shack, had just opened up only a mile from the hospital.

I perked up, exclaiming, "Oh, a burger would be amazing!"

Delighted to hear that I was finally hungry, they headed out immediately to get me a plain burger with nothing on it, in hopes that I could keep it down. But when they arrived at Shake Shack, the line to order was several blocks long. Apparently, we weren't the only ones who were excited not to have to go all the way to California for a Shake Shack burger.

By the time they came back an hour and a half later with the hard-won burger, I had lost my appetite and been consumed with nausea once again. I begged them to take the burger and fries out of my room, as the smell made me want to throw up.

Still, their devoted desire to help me regain the weight I had lost inspired me to try even harder over the following days.

I took tiny micro-steps forward, challenging myself to take one more swig of protein shake, to attempt a single bite of something solid, to breathe through the nausea, and try to keep my food down.

I reassured myself that even if I were only able to gain a few ounces, I would be stronger for surgery than when I arrived in Seattle. And although I was weak compared to my pre-sepsis self, I had never been stronger since surviving sepsis. I was learning, one moment at a time, to let go of unfair comparisons to a body that was no longer mine.

The million baby steps I'd taken in my recovery had prepared me for the giant step ahead. As scared as I was, I envisioned a future where I would walk again and live independently. I didn't know how I would get there, but I knew my leg surgery was the necessary next step.

The only way out is through.

CHAPTER 14

WALKING THROUGH FIRE

"The brave man is not he who does not feel afraid, but he who conquers that fear."

– Nelson Mandela

October 22, 2018 - The Big Day

Twenty-two is a significant number for me. Though my daughters were born in different months, they were both born on the 22nd, as was my brother Rick. When Jordan was born on the 22nd, nearly three years after her sister, 22 officially became our family's lucky number. Whenever it pops up in our lives – in a phone number, on a license plate, on a sports jersey, or wherever – we see it as a good omen.

Terrified as I was to lose my lower legs, when I learned my leg amputation surgery was scheduled for October 22nd, Rick's birthday, I took it as a positive sign. Like God saying, "Relax. I've got you."

With everything falling into place, I focused on the few things within my control. I had done all I could to physically prepare for surgery.

Now I had to mentally prepare to hand myself over to the surgeons who would remove my damaged feet, changing my body forever.

No Turning Back

I slept in a drug-induced slumber the night before my surgery and woke up groggy, unfocused on the sacrifice ahead. I kept my eyes closed and tried to rest as I was taken by gurney to the pre-op room in the basement of Harborview. Now that this day had arrived, my surgery couldn't come fast enough. I just wanted it behind me.

I had two requests on the day of surgery, suggested to me by a friend who'd been through a similar procedure. First, I didn't want to see any of the instruments they would be using. I didn't even want to imagine what they might be. Second, I wanted to be put under as quickly as they could get it done so that I could get through my surgery with as little psychological trauma as possible and focus on my recovery.

Because they followed those directives beautifully, I don't have much to share about the surgery itself. What I do remember is waking up afterward and realizing: *I did it! I did the hardest thing I've ever had to do! It's behind me, and I survived.*

The A-Word

Even after becoming an amputee, I still had a hard time using the words *amputation*, *amputate*, and *amputee*. But in the recovery room, when I first looked down and saw my shortened legs with my bed covers obscuring them, I started using those words in my head. I wasn't supposed to talk because of the vocal cord procedure I'd just undergone, so I repeated the same words over and over in my head.

I am an amputee. I had my lower legs amputated.

Then I would change the emphasis on the words: *"**I** am an amputee, I **am** an amputee. I am an **amputee**."* These words swirled in my head for days as I tried to get comfortable with my new identity. Little by little, as my voice strengthened, I would ease into saying them out loud.

Going into that surgery was like jumping off a cliff, knowing it was the only route to where I needed to go. It was terrifying and took courage to make that leap, but I knew I had to do it to move ahead. Now that my surgery was finally in the rearview mirror, I could move forward with my new life.

I was comfortable as they wheeled me back up to my room, where Dani, Jordan, and Scott were anxiously awaiting my arrival. I slept for a while, but awakened in overwhelming pain. The epidural I had been given as a pain blocker wasn't working for me. My pain would have to be managed with medication in my IV instead. The nurses warned that this meant my first couple of days post-surgery would be more difficult than anticipated. Frustrating news, but it was beyond my control, so I steeled myself for what lay ahead, reminding myself that my recovery was moving in the right direction.

As frail and helpless as I felt in my new body, as uncertain as I felt in my new identity as an amputee, and amidst all of the pain and fear, I sensed a flickering spark of strength I had never known before. I had just done the hardest thing I'd ever done in my life. I wasn't going to give up now. My goal moving forward was to do everything I could to help that flame grow.

Brother Rick and "Sister" Heidi

My brother Rick, and one of my oldest and dearest friends, Heidi, had been desperate to see me since I'd returned to Washington. They were both in Spokane, and Scott had been texting with them daily. He asked Rick to come help me immediately after my surgery, and asked Heidi to give me a few days to recover before she came so that I wouldn't be overwhelmed. Rick considered it a birthday gift to finally be by my side, while Heidi struggled to wait her turn.

Heidi and I had been inseparable through middle and high school, and though we inevitably went our separate ways, we stayed in touch over the years. Like sisters. Though we lived in different cities, we saw each other as often as we could, supporting each other through life's milestones: college graduations, weddings, the births of our kids, and the deaths of our grandparents. She couldn't imagine me going through something so traumatic without being there to support me, so on the day of my surgery, she left straight from work and made the five-hour drive from Spokane to Seattle. She planned to spend a few days at her sister's place so that she would be nearby if we needed any help.

Heidi sent me the sweetest text before my surgery. She said she had that feeling you get at the beginning of a relationship when you can't stop thinking about that person all day and night. She'd felt like this for the past month since she first heard about my sepsis-induced brush with death, and she couldn't wait to see me. I was so happy, knowing she was thinking of me and would be with me soon.

When she arrived in Seattle, realizing I had been out of surgery since earlier that day, she couldn't help herself. She went directly to the hospital and headed straight for my room. Not to go in, talk to, or disturb me in any way, just to peek in on me and reassure herself that I was okay.

As she exited the elevator on my floor, she saw two beautiful young women and their harried-looking father waiting at the elevator door.

They're here awfully late. I wonder if someone they love just had surgery too?

That's when she recognized Dani and Jordan, so much more grown-up than the last time she'd seen them, and realized who that exhausted father must be.

"Scott?" she called out. He looked up, and it took them both a moment to recognize the familiar set of eyes looking back at them from faces that had aged nearly 30 years since they'd last spent time together.

Scott reminded Dani and Jordan that this was Heidi, my bestie from Spokane. The girls had been texting with her for weeks and were delighted to see her in person. She and Scott hugged each other and cried for me, the girl they had both loved since we were all young. How had they gone from celebrating high school graduation and our wedding together to being there to support me through such a horrific trauma?

"I swear, I wasn't going to interrupt her rest. I just had to be close to her," Heidi sobbed.

"Of course you did," Scott smiled through his tears. "I wouldn't have expected any less from you."

The next day, with Scott's and my blessing, Heidi joined Rick and my family at my bedside for the first few days post-surgery. I was relieved to know that Rick was reporting back to my parents and my brother George, who were all anxious to hear about my recovery and were awaiting their chance to be near me. Although I was struggling to manage the pain and couldn't speak because of the surgery to my vocal cords, I was comforted to have them both nearby.

Pain, Pain, Go Away

The next few days were unbearable, despite everyone's best efforts to keep my pain under control. I was given a Patient-Controlled Analgesia (PCA) pump that allowed me to administer pain medication at the earliest safe interval, ensuring there was never a delay while waiting for a nurse. As soon as it was safe to take the next dose, I could push a button to release it directly into my bloodstream. Unfortunately, the meds were consistently wearing off before my next dose was due, leading to regular intervals of terrible pain, which I had no option but to endure. The nurses were right: an IV drip is *not* as effective as an epidural.

Whenever the pain returned, Rick, Scott, Heidi, or the girls would show me photos on their phones and distract me with stories about our lives together. They'd watch movies with me. At the same time, I sat with my thumb on the button, pushing it over and over until the next dose of medication was finally administered. Even after receiving the medication, it would be another 10 to 20 minutes before the pain would subside. I kept repeating my mantra and reminding myself that this level of pain shouldn't last for more than a few days.

In my most desperate moment, I remember being doubled over in pain with my eyes closed, crying for someone to get a nurse. Scott reminded me that I was in the home stretch, while Jordan thoughtfully took the controller from my hand, reassuring me that she would keep pushing the button for me. Dani went to the nurse's station and returned with a nurse armed with a dose of something to help me sleep, since I was already at the maximum dose of painkillers. With my eyes clenched shut, I kept repeating my mantra over and over until I dozed off, finally released from the relentless pain.

The only way out is through. The only way out is through. The only way out is through…

A Peek at my Future

I wasn't ready to look under the covers at my bare legs until the morning after my surgery, when I awoke with just Scott in my room. Still unable to speak, I wrote him a note saying I wanted to look at my legs before anyone else arrived. He helped me fold back my blankets, and together we looked at my shortened legs, wrapped securely in post-surgical bandages. We took in the reality that my feet were gone forever.

My emotions were conflicted: I was grieving for the loss of my feet, but also grateful for the surgery that had saved my life. Scott comforted me, rubbing my thigh to remind me that these were still my legs. They looked small and helpless, but they were still my legs.

Now that the surgery we had been anticipating for so long was complete, we could finally slow down and take some time to begin grappling with our complicated feelings about my amputations. I wrote Scott another note saying how sad I was that my life would never be the same. I was afraid I wouldn't be able to do many of the things I used to do, like yoga, walking on the beach, working out, cooking, traveling, and fully caring for myself. In my fragile state, that list seemed endless.

“I’m sad too,” he admitted, holding me close. He explained that, ever since I’d gotten sick, he’d been struggling with how unfair it was that something this traumatic had to happen to me. He felt helpless, unable to stop it from happening.

“But I’m so grateful you survived.” His eyes filled with tears as he promised that he and the girls would be with me through my recovery and into my future. They would help me relearn how to do the things I loved to do, with whatever adaptations I needed. He reminded me that Dani and Jordan had told him in the ICU that they knew I would want to survive, even if it meant losing my hands and feet. I had always talked about their weddings and my future grandkids and they knew I wouldn’t want to miss out on all that for any reason.

They were right. Even in the midst of my deep sorrow and loss, I was grateful to be alive.

I was also grateful that Scott felt safe enough with me to finally begin sharing how challenging all this had been for him. He had been under so much pressure to make sure everyone else was okay that he hadn’t had time to feel his way through his own conflicted emotions. Together, we were both learning to allow space for ourselves and each other to feel sorrow, along with the tremendous gratitude that I was still alive.

Finding my Voice

Two days after surgery, I was finally allowed to start talking. I was relieved to hear that my voice was no longer as hoarse as it had been, reassuring me that the surgery had been a success. I was testing out my new voice, telling Scott that I hadn’t slept well and was in much greater pain than I expected. Just then, a man I’d never met came into my room with his arms full of thick cotton batting and casting material.

He introduced himself as a member of the prosthetics team and told me he was there to put casts on my legs. He explained that the casts would protect the ends of my residual limbs as they healed and keep my legs straight, so my muscles wouldn't shorten. This would allow my knees to fully straighten once healed.

Immediately, my entire body clenched. As important as that sounded, I knew I was still in too much pain for something like that, but I didn't know if I had the right to say no. I decided that the worst that could happen was that he could say no to my no. So I spoke up.

"I know you came all this way," I began apologetically, "but I don't feel like I can do this today. My legs still hurt so much. If you touch them or move them in any way, it's just going to be unbearable for me. Even sitting still, I'm in so much pain right now."

I was surprised when he replied, "That's okay," with a warm smile and turned to leave. "I'm glad you let me know. I'm just one floor away. I'll check back in tomorrow."

I felt both relieved and empowered. I had used my new, stronger voice, and it had been respected. I was gaining back control of my life.

Caring for my Future

The next morning, Heidi was with us when an in-home caregiver recommended by a friend arrived for an interview. She was a few years older than me, very no-nonsense, and clearly qualified for the position. But frankly, after the parade of nurses and doctors who'd been in my personal space and up in my private business every moment since I'd arrived at the hospital, the idea of inviting yet another stranger into my home was overwhelming.

"So, what do you think?" Scott asked me after she'd left.

I shrugged, "She seems fine."

Heidi pulled Scott aside. "Can you hold off before you make a final decision? Katy didn't seem excited about this nurse, and they'll be spending a lot of time together. My mom knows a lot of people in the medical field and may know someone. I can check with her tonight."

Although he was eager to get that key decision squared away, Scott agreed. Clearly, I wasn't in the right frame of mind to make a decision that would affect my daily life in such an intimate way and for so long.

When Heidi asked her mom if she knew any caregivers, she realized why her gut had been telling her there was a better fit for me.

"You know, my friend Todd is a nurse," Heidi's mom reminded her.

"Oh my God, Todd! I love Todd!" Heidi laughed at the obvious oversight. "Of course! Do you think he's available?"

"I know he is. He just got back to town after a job in Palm Springs. He's been taking temporary nursing assignments while looking for a full-time position. He and Katy would love each other."

Heidi agreed. Todd was the perfect nurse for the job.

Todd

After a quick conversation with Scott, laying out Todd's credentials – nurse, experienced caregiver, long-time family friend, clean and sober – Heidi called Todd in for an interview.

Honestly, I was too overwhelmed with my time in the hospital to imagine my life at home. All I recall about that interview was that Todd seemed nice, and if Heidi trusted him, I trusted him too. So I left it up to Scott to make the final call.

"I'm going out to the waiting room to talk to Todd a bit more," Scott announced, gesturing out the door. The two of them stepped out into the hallway, leaving me in the room with Heidi, Dani, and my nephew Darrick, who had been visiting regularly since I arrived back in Seattle. Jordan had returned to school a few days after my surgery.

"I'm just not equipped to take care of her through this," Scott leveled with Todd, "I love her more than anything, but I'm not a caretaker."

"That's great," Todd told Scott, "I'm glad you know your place in this whole thing. You can't be everything to her, and you shouldn't try to be. She doesn't need you to take care of her; she needs you to keep loving her as you do, and to let me step in to handle her daily needs. That's what I'm here for."

Scott was sold. "Thank you. That was exactly what I needed to hear."

Back in the room, Scott told me, "Todd gets it. He's our guy."

That he was. Choosing Todd as my caregiver was one of the best decisions we made in the whole process, and I will always be grateful to Heidi for listening to her gut and bringing him into our lives. He brought a much-needed breath of fresh air into our battle-fatigued midst, helping us reclaim some of the joy we'd lost along the way. In the process, he enmeshed himself in our family in the most loving and seamless way possible. We will love him always.

Casting Call

By the third day post-surgery, my pain was finally becoming manageable. When the prosthetist returned for my casts, I agreed to do them on the condition that he would stop if my pain felt unbearable. He explained the process to me as he carefully wrapped my legs in cotton batting and gently applied the plaster casting material around my calves, up to the center of my thighs.

This was my first official prosthetist visit as an amputee. I had so many questions about the healing process, the type of physical therapy I should do to prepare my muscles to walk again, and the making of my first set of prosthetic legs. He carefully explained every step of the process and reminded me to focus on regaining the weight I had lost, working to build muscle in my upper body and core. I would get to work on my leg muscles in physical therapy as soon as my casts were permanently removed in a few weeks.

By the time he finished casting my second leg, I'd learned that I might have my first prosthetic legs as early as Christmas. If all went well, I might stand again before New Year's Eve!

All Clear for Take-off

Before I could leave the hospital, one nagging question had to be answered. My medical team needed to make sure a small mass on my liver that they'd seen on the scans was not causing me any complications. They suspected it was scar tissue from a benign cyst, but after all I had overcome, they weren't taking any chances. After a series of tests and close monitoring of my liver enzymes, we all breathed a collective sigh of relief when they ruled out anything serious.

Eight days after becoming an amputee, my appetite was finally returning, the pain in my legs was more manageable, and I was cleared for release. My family was overjoyed, but I had those same anxious feelings I'd had when my surgery was scheduled. I wasn't ready to leave the safety of the hospital.

That flame of strength was growing, but I still had my doubts. I had nearly died, lost both of my lower legs, and was being sent home with black fingertips, weighing 20% less than when I entered the hospital. For the past seven weeks, I'd had a team of nurses looking in on me around the clock, and a team of specialists focusing on every system in my body. How would my family replace that?

Scott looked me in the eye. He gently squeezed my frail shoulders and assured me he had it under control. "You'll be in good hands, I promise."

"Alright," I reluctantly agreed, "if you think we're ready, let's do this." I felt myself standing on yet another cliff, with no choice but to jump. I was scared, but I knew I had to keep moving forward.

The only way out is through.

CHAPTER 15

COMING HOME

"The most important thing a man can know is that, as he approaches his own door, someone on the other side is listening for the sound of his footsteps."

– Clark Gable

Our home on Mercer Island, where we'd lived before moving to Hawaii, was perched on an expansive lot on Lake Washington. This home, with its stunning view of the lake and a glimpse of downtown Seattle in the distance, held nostalgic memories of raising our daughters through their elementary school years, especially since Midori and her two boys, roughly the same age as Dani and Jordan, still lived next door.

We'd bought the house sight unseen almost 20 years earlier, when we found out through Midori that the family who'd owned it for over 30 years was about to sell it to a developer who planned to raze the house and build a McMansion. We had always loved the lake and sunset views when barbecuing at Midori's and dreamt about someday having a place on that side of the lake ourselves. Knowing how rarely houses in that neighborhood came up for sale, and that this house would get snatched up quickly if we didn't act immediately, we made a full-price offer that same night.

Though the house itself was obscured by the trees and shrubs separating it from Midori's, we were already well acquainted with the yard. The vast lawn that led down to the water from Midori's house was the mirror image of this yard, with no fence or landscaping separating them. Midori's upper yard had a large sports court, and the neighboring yard (now ours) had two big elm trees with a tire swing where the kids were allowed to play. Our girls had already spent countless hours in the park-like setting of the combined lawns.

It felt like serendipity that we were able to buy that house, allowing our girls to grow up in this idyllic setting on the lake next to two of their best friends. And that suburban village setup wasn't just great for our kids and us, it was mutually beneficial. After Midori and her husband separated, she became a single mother working full-time at Microsoft, and we were more than happy to help out with her boys as the kids joyfully, if chaotically, entertained each other.

All these years later, we were returning to our village to receive the support we needed in kind. With our collective kids grown up and living away from home, we knew that having Midori next door as an extra set of hands during my recovery would be a godsend.

Homecoming

On the day I left the hospital, as we drove up the street where my kids had learned to ride their bikes so many years before, I relished the colors of the changing fall leaves. It was something I always missed while living in Hawaii. My nostalgia turned to panic, however, as we turned down the steep driveway to our Mercer Island home. I couldn't imagine anyone would be able to push me up such a sharp incline in my wheelchair, or that I'd ever be able to walk on a steep hill like that again.

As we pulled into the garage, my dread shifted to the next terrifying task: transferring out of the car into my wheelchair. The occupational therapist had given me a little wooden slide to help ease the transition, but the seat in my SUV was much higher than the bed where I'd practiced, and I was worried that Scott and Dani wouldn't know how to help me. I had fretted about this the whole way home from the hospital after the awkwardness of getting me into the car in the first place.

I stared at my black fingertips, knowing how easily they could be injured, then looked past them to the big, cumbersome casts on my truncated legs. After suffering such terrible trauma, the visions my mind concocted were like something out of a horror movie. I imagined falling, breaking bones in my hands and legs, and reopening my surgical wounds. I worried I would instinctively reach my hand out to open the door, and my rigid fingertips would break off and fall to the garage floor. Things I formerly thought impossible had actually happened to me recently, so now it seemed like any horrific thing could occur at any time.

To make matters worse, memories of the years I had spent easily walking between the house and the garage were swirling through my head, steeping me in self-pity. I was embarrassed and angry as hot tears began to roll down my cheeks. I had never felt so helpless and out of control.

I knew I needed to get out of the car, but it seemed impossible. I was angry at Scott for wanting to bring me home so soon, certain we had made a mistake. Looking back, I'm sure he was afraid too.

Then I saw Todd, my new nurse, come out of the house to help. I had forgotten he would be there. Though I'd only met him briefly and we hadn't yet bonded, Heidi's love for him and his experience as a private nurse comforted me, and I felt my muscles begin to unclench.

As Todd opened my door to assist Scott, Dani confidently stepped in to assist as well. I could see that she was ready, willing, and able to help me with anything I would need in my new life. Scott and I wouldn't have to navigate my convalescence on our own. Between these three competent helpers, plus Midori next door, I had a dedicated, skilled nursing team taking care of me.

As anticipated, getting me out of the car was awkward, but Scott, Dani, and Todd each had at least one hand on me the whole time to ensure I wouldn't be injured. Scott opened the garage door, and Todd wheeled me outside. Dani carried vases of flowers, boxes of get-well cards, cozy blankets, and other gifts.

I felt safe in my wheelchair on the new ramp, which ran straight across the patio from the garage. I was relieved that the ramp wasn't sloped, and there were safety boards along the sides, creating a lip that kept my wheelchair from falling over the edge. It wasn't at all rickety or scary, as I had feared.

After expertly navigating the tall threshold separating the stoop from the kitchen, Todd wheeled me into the house where I had raised my kids a decade earlier.

I was immediately comforted by the smell of homemade soup simmering on the stove. The scent filled my mind with images of seven-year-old Jordan, ten-year-old Dani, and their friends running past me in the kitchen to go play down by the lake. I could see myself standing by the stove, stirring that pot of soup.

My vivid imagination was finally working in my favor, and I began to accept that this was again my home. As hard as it was for me to let go of all the things I could no longer control, the care that went into creating a safe, welcoming home for my family and me helped me relax and enjoy this homecoming.

I was surprised by how much the house felt the same as when we had lived there 10 years earlier. I couldn't believe how well-appointed and cozy it was. I was expecting temporary furnishings, but it looked like we had never left.

I saw an espresso maker, a toaster, and a complete set of knives sitting on the counter. A Halloween-themed dish towel I didn't recognize hung from the stove, and a few dirty dishes were piled up in the sink.

It hadn't really occurred to me until then that my family had been living here the whole time I had been at Harborview.

From the kitchen, I could look past the dining room and out the windows overlooking our backyard. Across Lake Washington, I could see Seattle. I had forgotten just how much I loved that view.

The water was calm, reflecting the clear sky above. Two tall elm trees in the center of our yard stood firm, virtually unchanged from the first time I had seen them years before. Looking at those elms daily over the coming months, I would begin to see them as a promise. Just like their sturdy trunks, my legs would one day stand tall and firm on the earth again. And just as those branches had once supported my kids while they swung happily back and forth on a swing that had long since been removed, I too would someday be able to support my family again, not just be supported by them.

The burnt sienna leaves carpeting the ground and the smattering of amber and burgundy leaves on the branches reminded me that I had arrived home at the changing of the seasons. Seattle was transitioning from summer to fall, signaling the city to slow down and prepare for renewal, just as I was.

I hadn't appreciated that change of seasons when I'd lived in Seattle before we moved to Hawaii, since fall leaves meant dark, rainy days were in store. But after living in the consistently hot days of Hawaii, I missed the rhythm of the seasons. The beauty of that fall day, as I returned to our home, reassured me that I was in the right place to heal and renew myself.

Looking past the kitchen, through the open dining and living area, I realized our old furniture had been replaced with similar pieces, making it feel instantly like home. Only the area rugs were missing, as the floors were thoughtfully left bare to ensure full wheelchair access. There was a new dining table where our old one used to be, covered with a beautiful pink French tablecloth. Dani told me she had chosen it for me, in memory of the trip we had taken to Paris together the prior spring.

Dani guided me into the living room and showed me a plush, white couch across from a gas fireplace. There was a brand-new TV hanging over it. She explained that they wanted this area to be especially comfortable for me, so I could recover in my own home while still being part of household activities. I could operate the TV, fireplace, and lights with remote controls, and I could easily communicate with people in the kitchen and dining room. When it came time to have guests over, two people could fit comfortably on the couch with me, and there were cozy chairs nearby, if needed. They had thought of everything.

Dani explained that while some of our friends and family helped move Midori's furnishings back to her house, others donated their spare furnishings to help transform our former house into this beautiful home. They even stocked the pantry, refrigerator, cupboards, bedrooms, and bathrooms with everything we would need while living there.

She was especially excited to show me my new accessible bedroom just off the living room. Sunlight streamed through the large corner windows onto a rented adjustable hospital bed with a view of a private garden. Next to the bed was a wheeled table that could swing over my bed or be pushed aside as needed. It was exactly like the one I had used in the hospital. This setup felt familiar and eased my transition home.

Down pillows and stuffed animals from friends sat on the soft pink bedspread, making the room feel cozy and comfortable. It reminded me of the floral childhood bedrooms I had once decorated for my girls in that same house.

Dani showed me a small wheelchair with a toilet seat that could be pushed over a regular toilet, so I wouldn't need to use a bedpan as I had for the past five weeks in the hospital. She demonstrated the controls on the bed, which could be raised or lowered to make my wheelchair transfers more comfortable, and showed me how easy it would be to sit up or lie back at any angle with the aid of the bed.

On the corner of the table sat a fresh bouquet of fall flowers, a salt lamp from a friend, and the diffuser for the essential oils that had helped me relax during my hospital stay. There was even a little pink bell, which Dani said I could use to summon help whenever I needed it. She reassured me that there would always be a helper nearby who would come right away when they heard the bell. She was easing all of my concerns about moving home.

The most striking and welcome addition to the room was the shower. Located in the corner, opposite the bed, it reminded me of a Fisher-Price playhouse made of thick, hollow plastic. It had a ramp on the front that Todd or Dani could use to push me up into it while I was sitting on the "toilet chair." The shower floor was about 18 inches off the ground, with a 3-foot wall that both provided privacy and prevented water from splashing onto the surrounding hardwood floors. It had a handheld shower that was connected to the sink in the adjacent powder room. Dani could stand outside and easily reach over the edge to help me as needed. I couldn't believe they found a way to get me my own shower! They truly had thought of everything.

I was thrilled at the prospect of finally taking a full shower and washing my hair. Until then, all my "baths" and rare hair washings had taken place in my hospital bed. My legs were too sore to plan a shower just yet, but I looked forward to the day when I would be well enough to wash my hair and body thoroughly. This would symbolize the true beginning of my recovery, putting my time in the hospital in my past.

Home is Where the Heart is

That first night back home, my nephew Darrick and his girlfriend came to help make dinner and carve pumpkins with Dani. I had always loved making holidays memorable for my kids with decorations and fun activities. Now, my family was making this holiday special for me.

Todd left for dinner with his husband, Michael, so we could settle into the house on our own. I was fretful as he left, but everyone assured me that he would return in a few hours to help me get through my first night at home. They promised he would stay overnight as often as I needed him.

The kids made dinner while I sat with Scott on my cozy new couch, watching Darrick's puppies play. I was sad to leave my dog, Olive, behind in Hawaii, and I loved being around the warm love of dogs again. They made it feel like home.

Just as we had done years earlier when we lived in that house, Dani put a classic Halloween movie on in the background while the kids carved pumpkins. Although Jordan wasn't with us, she called to welcome me home and sent photos from the Halloween dance she'd attended with Kai and her friends at school. It was the first time in weeks that my life felt somewhat normal.

By the time Todd returned, I was exhausted. It had been a long, emotional day. He helped me transfer into my wheelchair and took me to the bathroom, then changed me into a soft pajama top, a gift from a friend. We worked together on our first big challenge: figuring out how I could best get into bed from my wheelchair. Thankfully, my upper body was strong enough to help as he lifted me into my bed and settled me in.

My legs were extremely sore and cumbersome with their bulky casts. No matter what I did to reposition my body, it was impossible to get comfortable in plaster casts reaching up to my thighs. Fortunately, I had been sent home with strong painkillers and pills that would help me sleep. As Todd left my room, he promised he would set alarms on his phone and wake me up as needed to administer my medications without me having to worry about a thing. I was so relieved to be back in my house with Todd and my family watching over me.

Now that I was home, with a fabulous care team nearby, I could put my weeks in the hospital behind me. It was time to settle into my new normal. If there was one thing I had learned over the prior six weeks fighting for my life, it was that I wasn't doing any of this alone. My friends and family were making sure of that.

CHAPTER 16

FINDING COMFORT IN THE UNCOMFORTABLE

"Life begins at the end of your comfort zone. So if you're feeling uncomfortable right now, know that the change taking place in your life is a beginning, not an ending."

– Neal Donald Walsch

The first couple of weeks back in Seattle were deeply challenging. I had to accept that much of my life was beyond my control and try to find comfort in the midst of this unsettling state. I got through this time by reminding myself that I would feel a little bit better with each passing day and would eventually make significant improvements.

It was still hard to imagine a day when I would feel like my old self again, but I held out hope, focusing on the present and what I could control. I learned to be patient, to face my days one moment at a time, to lean on others, to accept all the help I was offered, and to ask for help when I needed it. Thank God for the many people who showed up.

The Wind beneath My Wings

"When I was a boy, and I would see scary things in the news, my mother would say to me, 'Look for the helpers. You will always find people that are helping.'"

– Fred Rogers

While still in Harborview, when I began to feel better after my amputations, Dani showed me a text chain that included about 15 of our closest friends and family in the Seattle area. Someone had sweetly changed the group name to "Katy's Krew." The texts began while I was still in the ICU on Oahu. Dani, Scott, Jordan, and Midori had formed the group as a special support network of my closest friends and family to help us in the coming months.

Along with a few other friends, the members of Katy's Krew had helped Dani and Midori set up our home on Mercer Island to accommodate my needs when I arrived. They also volunteered to help with meals and visited frequently, helping us feel less alone during our transition back to Seattle.

Knowing I had an entire team dedicated to easing my recovery was humbling and made me feel so supported. But I also struggled with feeling guilty that so many people were going out of their way for me.

"Mom, people really want to help," Dani reassured me. "They feel helpless, not knowing what they can do to make this easier for our family. When your friends heard you were coming back to Seattle, we got dozens of offers to help in any way we needed. Midori said she could get the house set up before we arrived if other friends could take on essential tasks. And they did. Robin loaded the refrigerator with condiments, meals, fruits, drinks, milk, and anything she thought we would need. Vicki did the same with the pantry, filling it with healthy snacks and any staples we might want over the coming months. A big group of people volunteered to help move Midori's things out of the house, and several families donated furnishings for the bedrooms and the rest of the house. They accomplished so much more than we ever expected, and they were happy to help."

There were another six to eight people in Katy's Krew who continually checked in and volunteered to visit regularly. They were among the group that furnished our home and made it accessible for my wheelchair, helped cook and clean, ran errands, went shopping, and made sure we knew we were never alone. Together with the dozens of others who brought lunches and dinners or chatted with me for hours, I had a fantastic support group for whom I will be forever grateful.

And that was just the beginning. For the next six months, we would receive fully cooked dinners three times a week until I was ready to resume cooking. I had regular visitors to break up the monotony of my days. Friends and extended family visited often from out of town to spend time with me and even to help care for me on a few occasions when Scott had to be gone overnight. I received dozens of cards and frequent flower deliveries.

I learned a lot about the reciprocity of giving and receiving. When I thanked everyone for all that they were doing for me, I was assured over and over again that they were grateful to have a way to help us through such a difficult time. I realized the best way to reciprocate their love was to accept their generosity as graciously as it was given.

Nurse Todd

Although he was new to our lives, Todd was a key member of Katy's Krew. My first week post-surgery, he worked around the clock to help with middle-of-the-night medications and trips to the bathroom. He slept in a spare bedroom that Dani had made up for him. Scott set up walkie-talkies so I could easily reach him during the night if I needed anything between my scheduled pills.

Todd greeted me in the mornings, assisted me with brushing my teeth, took me to the toilet, and helped me change into clean clothes. He'd then take me out to join Scott and Dani for coffee and breakfast at our windows overlooking the lake.

My pain was still intense enough the first few days that Todd had to set alarms throughout the night to wake me up before my pain pills wore off. Most of the time, he got to me before I needed him, but I was glad we had the walkie-talkies on the rare occasions when I had to ask for medication because the pain was unbearable. He was able to balance Tylenol with my heavy pain medications so they wouldn't wear off at the same time, but that meant waking up several times a night to take pills.

Todd would stay with me and tell me stories or ask me questions to keep my mind off the pain while we waited for it to subside enough that I could sleep. We were both exhausted, but like soldiers at war, those tough first nights together helped us bond quickly.

The intensity of my leg pain reminded me of labor pains. In an attempt to make it bearable between painkillers, I used the breathing techniques I'd learned from Lamaze and yoga. I would meditate by focusing on every deep breath and slow exhale to take my mind off the pain. The more I could focus on my breathing, the less the pain bothered me.

The nights were the most challenging part of my recovery; they reminded me of my time in the hospital. Alone in the dark with my thoughts, I worried obsessively and wept for the loss of my lower legs. To distract myself, I listened to music and podcasts as I drifted off to sleep. I couldn't bear to think about my situation.

Family and Friends

In addition to my immediate family, Scott's and my extended families did all they could to support us.

Early in my recovery, Scott and Dani arranged for Holly to visit from Utah because Todd would be taking the weekend off, and I was still in a lot of pain. I've known Holly since I was 16 because our husbands are brothers. She made our wedding cake, and I was invited to be at the birth of her second daughter. She's like a big sister to me. I've always felt safe with her.

Holly volunteered immediately when she heard we needed help. She was anxious to see how I was doing, since I was barely stable and not thinking clearly at all the last time she saw me. I didn't know it at the time, but when Holly came to Hawaii to be with me in the ICU, she had been visiting her daughter Eliza, in Seattle. She'd had to cut that trip short to be with us, so on this trip to Seattle, she would be able to make up some of that lost time with Eliza as well as help care for me. Having her and Eliza with us was like a ray of sunshine brightening our days.

Amazingly, Holly's visit was just the beginning. Over the next few months, we had relatives and close friends visiting from all over the country: my parents and brothers from Eastern Washington, my cousins from Montana, my best friends from Kauai and The Big Island, my aunt from Portland, and friends from Alaska, Texas, and New York. Some stayed at the house when we needed help, and others just visited when they were in town. Everyone lifted my spirits and kept my mind off my loss.

My friends from Seattle stepped up to help us with day-to-day things, and others visited when they could – some I had seen in the hospital, and others I hadn't seen since my school days.

One of my oldest friends, Kyle, visited from Australia. I hadn't seen him since college. He had been my graduation escort at our tiny high school in the early 80's. We reminisced about our time together at school and bonded over the shared experience we both had of nearly losing our lives.

Kyle had open-heart surgery when we were in 6th grade. I was terrified for him; open-heart surgery wasn't something I imagined happening to a 12-year-old. That was probably the first time in my life that I realized that someone I cared about could die.

I was so happy when he came back to school and was living proof that a person could survive something life threatening and fully recover. I remember him being less active for a while, but he was still the same smart, funny guy he had always been. He showed me that with perseverance, the human body can recover from even the most serious trauma.

As we sat in my living room forty years later, it felt good to share stories with a kindred spirit and celebrate the time with our families that we were both lucky to have.

My months of recovery allowed me to spend quality time with most of my extended family and friends from Hawaii, as well as a few other friends from afar. I count these many visits among the greatest blessings of this difficult period in my life.

Midori

Having Midori right next door was a great comfort to all of us, especially in those early days. Just knowing she was there, should we ever need her, allowed us all to relax. This was especially true in the evenings when Todd was off duty. She made a habit of checking in each morning and afternoon to see if any of us needed anything.

Having one of my best friends so nearby helped me keep loneliness and hopelessness at bay. Knowing that Midori was just a text away helped me feel less isolated during that largely homebound period of my recovery.

Cody

A surprise member of Katy's Krew and an unexpected superstar in my recovery was Midori's 12-year-old dog, Cody. He was a small, black-and-white Havanese I had known since he was a puppy. We never had an especially tight bond, though, because I lived so far away most of his life. He was around in the summers when I visited, but if Midori or her boys were nearby, he wasn't particularly interested in me.

That all changed when I arrived home after my leg amputations. This little mop of a dog became one of my most dedicated supporters. He could sense how much I needed extra love and care and became my constant recovery companion.

Cody first visited with Midori when she checked in on me after I arrived home from the hospital. She brought him along to see if I was comfortable around him with my sore legs and damaged fingers. When he saw me on the couch, he hopped up next to me, and I lifted him into my lap, where he curled up and let me pet him with my awkward fingers.

From that day forward, he made it his mission to snuggle up in my lap like it was his nine-to-five job, but without fanfare, as though this was something he had always done. That first day, I assumed it was just excitement because he hadn't seen me in a while, but it was more than that. Cody would be by my side for months, until he felt I was ready to manage life on my own.

It's hard to find a photo during this time when Cody isn't on my lap in my wheelchair, or sleeping next to me on the couch. If I snuck off while he was asleep, I would inevitably turn around to find him looking up at me with a betrayed expression. He would whine to be lifted into my wheelchair, knowing he couldn't make the jump himself. If nobody were around to help him onto my lap, he would follow me around until I returned to the couch, where he could safely reach my lap on his own.

Even when Midori and her boys visited me, I was the person Cody insisted on being near. Nothing about my situation scared him. He wasn't afraid of my wheelchair, and my constant movements to get comfortable didn't bother him at all. He would sit on my lap while I watched movies, had visitors, or talked on the phone, and insisted on riding with me in my wheelchair wherever I went. He was on my lap while I ate and when I visited with friends and family. He would even try to go into the bathroom with me! If I made him wait outside the bathroom door, I could hear him scratching and whining until I came out. Todd or someone else would gently lift him back onto my lap, where he would contentedly resume his duties as my emotional support Cody.

"Do you want to go see Katy?"

Midori texted me a video she'd recorded a few days into my recovery, showing Cody looking up into the camera and dancing excitedly. "Do you want to go see Katy?" she sang. He kept whipping his head toward the door and then looking back at her, prancing and whimpering excitedly.

When she said, "Okay, let's go," you could hear Cody's little toes scraping across the wood floor as he ran to her back door, which leads to my patio and kitchen. Cody then looked up at her exuberantly, dancing in circles while she unlocked and opened the back door. He immediately ran across her side yard, onto my patio, and up the steps leading to my kitchen, where he scratched on my door and waited impatiently for Todd to let him in.

This was the beginning of a daily routine that often included a phone call from Midori asking if Cody was at our house because she'd let him out her back door to go potty, and he'd disappeared. By the time she called, he was always sitting comfortably in my lap.

Midori would take Cody home for the night when she came to check in on how my day had been. This went on for months.

I don't know how he knew how much I needed him, but I'm so glad he did. He reminded me of the service dogs at the hospital, like Ipo, who came to visit me and my family while I was so sick. They were sweet and calm when they jumped up to lie beside me on my bed, letting me pet them or gently resting their heads on my thighs, comforting me with their warmth.

Cody also helped me keep my mind off Olive, our one-year-old "poi dog" (mixed-breed), who had stayed behind on Kauai. She was being cared for by friends until I was well enough to have a large, energetic dog back in the house with me. Although I missed her terribly, I knew I couldn't be around her; my legs and hands were still so fragile, and she was young and full of energy. Cody was a comforting distraction from her absence.

One day in January, after my surgeries had healed and I got my prosthetic legs, Cody suddenly lost interest in me and went back to spending his days at his own house. It was incredible to witness both his instinct to care for me when I needed his comfort and his intuitive understanding of when I would be fine without him.

My Mental Health

Once I made it past the most physically painful part of my leg amputation recovery, I began seeing a therapist. She helped me manage my complicated feelings about nearly dying and becoming an amputee, and supported me in dealing with the many ways it had changed my life. When I told her I felt helpless, she convinced me that all I had to do to regain some control was to ask to be included in decisions.

She encouraged me to start small, and as I gained confidence in my abilities, I could become increasingly more involved in decisions regarding my life. I would see her over the next few years as she helped me regain control of my future. With her guidance and encouragement, I gradually took on more responsibility for how I spent my time. Just as I had to trust others to make choices about my life in the hospital, I now had to begin trusting myself and my own decisions. I still relied heavily on my family and doctors, but I was starting to provide input on my life and recovery, helping me gain confidence that I would one day be taking care of myself again.

A Day in My New Life

"Patience is not passive. It is concentrated strength."

– Bruce Lee

Just like in the hospital, having a daily routine at home was essential. It made this overwhelming time more manageable by allowing me to focus on one thing at a time and provided consistency to keep my stress levels low. I constantly repeated the mantra, *one tiny step at a time,* to remind myself to focus on what was right in front of me rather than spinning out about a distant future I couldn't control.

I divided my daily schedule into a series of tasks, each split into tiny steps I mentally checked off as I completed them. Dividing my day into these bite-sized pieces made it bearable for me as my body slowly healed. This mental process allowed me to get through the monotony of months of recovery without becoming overwhelmed.

A typical day:

1. Morning routine
2. Breakfast
3. Talking with Dani or watching a movie or TV show on the couch
4. Taking my mid-morning medications
5. More TV, simple exercises, or a doctor's appointment
6. Lunch, often with a friend
7. Afternoon nap
8. Time with family
9. Dinner
10. Bedtime routine

Morning Routine

Mornings were challenging. Every morning, I had to come to terms with the reality that my lower legs had been amputated and my fingers were nearly useless because of the damaged tissue that had not yet been removed. Waking up felt like the movie *Groundhog Day*, where Bill Murray's character awakens every morning to the realization that he's reliving the same day over and over again. Likewise, I was faced with the daily reality that the nightmare that haunted me wasn't a dream: I had lost my lower legs to sepsis and would be losing my fingertips soon.

On top of that, I usually hadn't slept well because of severe pain and discomfort. I woke up nearly every hour throughout the night, continually disappointed that it wasn't morning, when I could spend time with my family. In the middle of the night, I would ruminate on negative thoughts. This made my situation seem unbearable, and I couldn't fall back asleep.

I eventually took the clock out of my room because it was constantly disappointing me; I would awaken to find I had only slept for an hour, or it would confirm that I had been awake in the middle of the night for an hour or more. I was always relieved when I woke to light streaming through my window and voices coming from the living room, signaling it was time to get out of bed and begin my day.

It was comforting to hear the people I loved talking and laughing together. Hearing Dani's voice always felt special, reminding me of times when the girls visited us over the holidays or during the summer when they were home from college. Even though I was awakening as an amputee and coming to terms with my new identity each morning, I was quickly reminded that I was surrounded by the people I loved.

Before sepsis, I would wake up each morning to the smell of brewing coffee, excited to start my day. I would hop out of bed, brush my teeth, quickly change into comfortable clothes, and head to the kitchen to make a latte before meeting Scott on our deck to enjoy the beautiful Hanalei view. I had always loved early mornings.

I felt that same craving when I woke up as a new amputee, but each day I was confronted with the fact that I could no longer rush through my morning routine and race out to my first latte. The pace of my life had changed, which was frustrating. I knew I had no choice but to accept it, though, since it would be my reality for the rest of my life.

One tiny step at a time.

On a typical day, I would ring my bell, and Todd would come in with a big smile and warm greeting to get me ready to join Scott and Dani for breakfast. I was usually due to take my morning pills. If my legs were still sore and we were waiting for the pain pills to kick in, he would open my blinds, straighten up my medicine tray, and pull up my sheets like he was tucking me in. He'd bring me a toothbrush and a hairbrush so I could brush my teeth and hair in bed.

As soon as I felt well enough, Todd would help me change into a clean shirt and loose shorts or sweatpants, then lift me off the bed and into the wheelchair. As I grew stronger, Todd did less of the heavy lifting as I learned how to get myself in and out of my bed and wheelchair with minimal help. Our simple routine could take half an hour or more, so I was constantly reminding myself to stay focused on the next step.

My mental checklist of steps looked something like this:

- Wake up
- Raise the back of my bed to sit up
- Ring for Todd
- Assess my pain level
- Greet Todd
- Take meds, if needed
- Brush teeth
- Brush hair
- Get dressed
- Move to the bathroom wheelchair
- Use bathroom
- Transfer to my regular wheelchair
- And so on

These tiny steps made my days bearable. I could easily complete each task, which gave me a much-needed sense of accomplishment and kept me out of my head, where I could become overwhelmed by my future.

One tiny step at a time.

After all that hard work, I was rewarded with my favorite part of the day: breakfast with Scott and Dani. Looking at the beautiful view out our corner picture windows, drinking a delicious latte, and feasting on the fruit, eggs, toast, or pastries that Todd served us every morning, reminded me of the breakfasts I always loved when traveling in Europe or staying in fancy hotels with Scott and the girls, or my closest friends. It was such a comforting way to start my days.

I could tell Todd understood how much breakfast meant to me; it showed in the artful way he presented even simple dishes like fanned apple slices in yogurt. His flair for hospitality helped lift my spirits, reminding me of the small pleasures in life and my gratitude that I was still alive to cherish them.

On the Couch

Never underestimate the importance of a fabulous couch when your mobility is impaired. Mine was the plush, white, designer sofa a friend with impeccable taste had given us. It was in the perfect location, smack-dab in the middle of our house, where I could see the beautiful view of the lake, and be seen while also seeing everything going on around me. Others could easily keep an eye on me and join me when they had time to chat or watch a special show with me.

I spent countless hours on that couch, resting, napping, chatting with visitors, and watching different TV series and movies with my family and friends as my body slowly healed. It seems silly to have fallen in love with a couch, but it kept me so comfortable and provided a central spot in my home, allowing me to be part of my loved ones' lives.

Morning Medications

Pills are a daily reality in recovery. Pills of varying shapes, sizes, and colors must be taken at all hours of the day and night. Keeping them all straight, taking them at the right time and in the right way, and managing the side effects is challenging enough. Layer on top of that anxieties about a family history of addiction, and you have a recipe for significant struggle. But since the alternative was mind-bending pain, I learned to accept and manage the process, with a lot of help from my family and nurse Todd.

I was privileged to be able to entrust my weekday medication management to Todd, a trained professional who made sure I got enough to keep me functional without becoming dependent. With his help, my family and I learned how to manage my schedule at night and on days when he wasn't working. When it came time to lower my doses and eventually stop using the more addictive pills, Todd and my doctors taught me how to manage the tapering process safely. Todd checked in with me regularly to be sure I still needed the most potent painkillers and helped me wean off of them as soon as I was able.

Even with Todd's help, it was a challenge. After all I had been through, I was loath to do anything that could lead to more pain. And the narcotics not only numbed my physical pain, but they numbed the emotional pain as well. As I gained more mental clarity when my doses were lowered, the reality of having parts of my body taken from me weighed much more heavily on my heart.

It scared me to realize that if my family and Todd hadn't been holding me accountable for taking my medications responsibly, I would have been tempted to stay on them longer and might have had difficulty getting off them. My heart goes out to anyone who is struggling with addiction.[1]

Exercises and Appointments

Daily exercise was essential, not only to help me recover but also to remind me that my body could still be strong and reliable, even though it was different from what it had been. Physical therapy was therapeutic beyond the physical, helping to keep depression and anxiety at bay.

All my daily movement felt like exercise as I got used to my new body, but we also found creative ways to keep me moving and break up the tedium of the endless leg lifts and clamshells my physical therapists

---

1. If you or someone you love is struggling to get off of a prescribed medication, resources are available. Here's a good place to start: https://www.samhsa.gov/find-help/helplines/national-helpline

prescribed. My niece set up TRX cables for me to strengthen my upper body and core. We also got an immersive virtual reality (VR) game console that I could play while sitting on the couch or in my wheelchair, to challenge my mind and body and get me out of my usual surroundings for a bit. The games were carefully chosen to suit my abilities. It was freeing to immerse myself in a fantasy world, stimulating my mind while working on hand and arm coordination and upper body balance.

Still, VR can't compare with actual outings. Though leaving the house was always a bit scary in this new incarnation, it was worth the trouble just to feel like part of the world again. Having regular appointments with my medical care team was important not just for my physical health but also for my mental well-being. Those check-ins allowed me to interact with people outside my home and created weekly and monthly routines that fit into my daily schedule. It was empowering knowing that each appointment was slowly moving my recovery forward.

Those appointments also offered a regular opportunity to practice navigating in a wheelchair in a setting designed to accommodate people with diverse physical abilities. With Todd's help, I learned how to use my new disability parking pass to park close to entrances and found accessible buttons to open doors, as well as elevators and ramps, to avoid stairs.

My Other Voices

Both Todd and Scott were incredible advocates for my care. I couldn't speak well on my own behalf, not only because my vocal cords were still recovering, but also because the painkillers numbed my mind and limited my understanding. Despite my efforts to stay positive, I was having difficulty believing I would eventually recover. I was constantly battling the fear that I would be in a wheelchair and in pain for the rest of my life, and would be unable to adapt to the loss of my fingers and feet. I was afraid that I would never again think clearly. I needed Todd and my family to help me plan for a future that, in my mind, was just a pipe dream.

Scott always came to my first appointment with each new doctor, therapist, and prosthetist to ensure nothing was overlooked. He made sure they fully understood my situation and all the ways sepsis had affected my health, both physically and mentally. He wanted to set the stage so I would get the treatments I needed to get back to a semblance of my prior active life. Todd was responsible for accompanying me to my ongoing medical appointments and relaying any pertinent information to the rest of the family.

We had a big calendar on which Todd, Dani, and Scott wrote color-coded notes. Todd had a color for my medical appointments; Dani used a different color to keep track of the people dropping off dinners. She also had an eye-catching, bright pink pen she would use for visits from friends and family. Just seeing that tell-tale pink on the calendar gave me an instant mood boost, knowing that a loved one would be visiting soon.

Lunch Dates

Amidst my struggles with pain and sorrow about my amputations, friends were constantly showing up to help in any way they could. As word spread, more and more of my Seattle friends reached out to visit me. I had always enjoyed going out for lunch or coffee with friends, so Dani set up two to three lunch dates a week, inviting friends over and asking them to bring enough food for four, so that Todd and my family could eat as well. Todd would artfully arrange the lunches on plates and serve my friend and me, and the rest of the food would be divided among my caretakers. It was a brilliant system because it resulted in a variety of lunches to keep my days more interesting, and it took the task of shopping and cooking for that day off the proverbial plates of Dani and Todd.

My family knew I would enjoy the social interaction, and it gave them time to focus on their own lives. It made me feel like the belle of the ball because so many people I had known over the years wanted to see me. They came to offer love and support, and to hear all I had been through and how I was feeling. They also came to enjoy a nice meal with an old friend. These lunches helped me remember that, despite all I had suffered and how my life had changed, I was still me.

I loved spending time with my friends in person, thanking them for everything they had done to support my family and me during this difficult time. The overwhelming love in our hearts, buoyed by their tremendous support, helped us through the pain and loss.

Afternoon Nap

Never underestimate the power of a good nap. To have the energy for quality time with my family in the evening after the morning's activities, the afternoon nap was a must. I didn't always sleep long, or even at all, but having that downtime built into my schedule to rest, relax, and recuperate was nonnegotiable. This afternoon siesta habit has stayed with me for years.

Dinner

Each weekday, Todd would set us up for success with dinner prep, then take his leave for the evening or weekend. Dinner was an extension of family time, and I had the pleasure of watching my family step up and take on the joys and challenges of cooking and cleaning.

Todd also did meal planning and shopping. If I didn't have a doctor's appointment on his shopping days, he would take me with him to the grocery store. Our local gourmet grocery store was, hands down, my favorite venue for an outing. It was my Disneyland. There was so much to see, interact with, and experience. Not just the food, but the people too.

At the grocery store, I felt like my old self again. I was shopping as I always had, helping plan meals and buy the foods I wanted at home. There was a sense of camaraderie, or at least commonality, with the other shoppers. It made me feel like I belonged and gave me a larger sense of community.

Bedtime Routine

After dinner, it fell to either Scott or Dani to help me with my bedtime routine. I cherished this time with them. They would take me through each step until I was safely in bed and ready for sleep, then they carefully laid out nighttime pills in little paper cups before they left. I would set a medicine alarm for the middle of the night and hope it would wake me before the pain did. My little pink bell sat by my bedside in case I needed help during the night.

Lather, rinse, repeat.

One tiny step at a time.

CHAPTER 17

WALKING BACK INTO THE FIRE

"When Alice fell down the rabbit hole, it was an accident, but when she stepped through the looking glass, it was of her own free will, and a braver deed by far."

– *Alice in Wonderland*, by Lewis Carroll

Skin and Bones

After my first few medical appointments, once Scott had met everyone on my team, Todd and I went to my many appointments at Harborview on our own. He and I were bonding, and our relationship felt more natural day by day. I felt safe in his care and comfortable having him by my side as we navigated my new world.

I'll never forget the first appointment when they removed my casts to replace them with new ones. It was the first time I was able to see my amputated legs since they had begun to heal. I was wearing jean shorts, and my legs were so skinny I could see the outline of my bones in my pale thighs. My knobby knees – one still bearing the scars of my fall on the bathroom stairs in Kauai when I was unknowingly tumbling down the sepsis rabbit hole – led down to swollen calves and the red, healing incisions where my legs had been amputated.

My emotions were jumbled. I was grateful for the brief opportunity to see my legs for a few minutes before fresh casts were put on them, but it was eerie to see my actual skin and bones ending where I once had ankles and feet. The dichotomy between the cute denim shorts I had always loved wearing and my sickeningly skinny legs, which now ended halfway down my calves, was baffling. I had the hardest time believing this was my actual body. It seemed so unreal.

I took photos to send to my daughters and parents. I wanted to give them the same opportunity I now had to come to grips with the reality of what my body had become. But I also wanted them to see that, beneath those casts, I still had part of my lower legs, and that my body was healing well despite being depleted by all I had been through.

Losing my Grip

A month after my leg amputations, and two months after going into septic shock, I returned to Harborview to have my seven black fingertips amputated. We gave Todd the day off so that Scott and I could have some time alone to process and prepare for this surgery. Scott woke me up at five a.m. to help me get dressed for the final surgery needed to put the worst of the sepsis trauma behind me. I put on the clothes Todd and I had laid out the night before: comfortable sweatpants and a loose T-shirt that would easily fit over my bandaged hands once my surgery was complete.

Because of the many nerves in my fingers, I was especially dreading these amputations. As hard as I tried not to worry about it, my mind was filled with doubts. The pain and discomfort of my leg recovery had been almost unbearable. What if the pain in my fingers was worse?

I use my hands to do so many things. Even with the black fingertips, I still waved my hands around when I spoke and grabbed things without thinking. What if I injured my fingers while they were healing? Or worse yet, what if I lost motor function in my hands after the surgery? I couldn't handle any more loss.

It was agonizing to make myself go in for yet another surgery. My old mantra came back to me: *The only way out is through.* Once this surgery was behind me, I would be in the home stretch. All I had to do was get through it.

As I had done so many times before, I focused on each of the steps I needed to complete to get through the surgery, trying not to think about the day ahead. I knew worrying about something I couldn't control was fruitless, so whenever my mind wandered to the what-ifs, I refocused on whatever task was next. We went methodically through our morning routine, skipping breakfast because of the surgery, and headed to the car with the promise of soon putting my surgeries behind us for good.

When we arrived at the hospital, we parked in our usual spot and took the underground walkway to the waiting room for the surgical suites in the adjacent building. Scott pushed my wheelchair down the long hospital corridor we regularly took to my leg appointments, but this time was different from the many times I had traveled this route before. Rather than taking the elevator to another floor, I was heading straight back into the surgical suite where my legs had been amputated.

I could feel the pit in my stomach growing as we got closer, aware with every step Scott took as he pushed my wheelchair that time was passing and my surgery was getting closer. Coming back to Harborview from the safety of my home to have this surgery was more emotionally challenging than my leg surgery had been. The first surgery felt like an inevitable extension of my hospital stay, but now here I was, coming back to the hospital of my own free will, volunteering to have my fingertips surgically removed. I kept feeling a panicked urge to change my mind, turn around, and leave.

But I knew this surgery was something I had to do; I only had to look down at my hands to be reminded that my black fingertips couldn't be saved. Though I'd gotten used to navigating the world with dead, brittle fingertips, it was challenging. Imagine if the ends of your fingers were made out of thick twigs – how cumbersome and frustrating it would be to pick things up, eat, write, apply makeup, use a phone, or do anything you need to get done. Now imagine you can never take them off because *they are your fingers*. Worse still, should one of those twigs break, you'd be at risk of infection, not to mention deeply traumatized by the fact that *one of your fingers just broke off.* It sounds dramatic, but this could actually happen if I didn't get the surgery soon.

Amputation was the only option. I knew that. But knowing that and accepting it were two different things.

As we approached the surgical check-in area, I closed my eyes and took four deep, slow breaths… in through my nose and out through my mouth, as I relaxed the muscles in my body. I said a silent prayer for a successful surgery and a speedy and painless recovery. I asked for complete healing, physical strength, and the ability to handle all of the changes in my life. I prayed that I would walk comfortably again and use my hands functionally.

I don't remember getting ready for surgery after my prayer, although I remember telling the pre-op team once again that I wanted to be sedated immediately. And just like last time, the next thing I remember is waking up in the recovery area, my finger surgery behind me.

On the Other Side

I felt no pain as I scanned my body, trying to feel if the surgery had been completed. There was a woman in recovery next to me who had family visiting, and I listened to them chatting while I lay there, too drowsy to open my eyes. I could feel Scott rubbing my arm and I knew I was safe. I was afraid to move my hands for fear of pain. I had been hyperaware of all of the nerve endings in my fingertips since I first felt the pain of DIC over two months earlier. I was in no rush to feel that pain again.

I opened my eyes to see Scott by my side, his hand resting gently on my leg. We gave each other a weak smile, happy the surgery was behind us, but also well aware of the impending pain and tough recovery ahead. When I was more alert, a transport person arrived to take me to the room where I would spend one night, before returning home.

Scott escorted my gurney up to the room, which looked like every other hospital room I had stayed in throughout this experience. Memories flooded in. I flashed through a slideshow of images of the emergency department on Kauai, waking up in the ICU at Queen's, seeing my blackened fingertips and purple hands and then my damaged feet, riding on a gurney down to the hyperbaric chamber, being wrapped like a burrito in preparation for my airlift to Seattle, and coming to Harborview for my leg surgery. What a whirlwind the last two months had been.

As I felt my anxiety rising, I closed my eyes and began doing the breathwork I had learned to help my body relax. I reminded myself that I was safe, I had an incredible medical team along with my loving family and friends supporting me, I was strong and could get through this, and all of my surgeries were now behind me. I could finally focus solely on my recovery. I began to feel a sense of relief seep into my body.

I'm sure Scott was experiencing similar post-traumatic stress being back in a hospital room by my side. He didn't show it, though, because he was being strong for me. I knew he was taking it day by day, moment by moment, and using breathing exercises and prayer to get through this difficult time, just as I was.

He gallantly spent the night in my hospital room, sleeping on an uncomfortable chair designed to pull out like a tiny bed. He'd done the same thing through both of my c-sections and many nights while I was at Queen's. I'm sure it was a relief to know this was the last night he'd have to do this for a very long time.

I slept comfortably, waking up only once to see a nurse changing an IV bag at my bedside. Whatever they gave me for the pain was helping me sleep better than I had since my life had been transformed by sepsis. I welcomed a night where this whole nightmare faded away.

I awoke in the morning to find Scott drinking coffee, preparing for our departure from the hospital. He explained that a nurse had been in to check on me and was waiting for the doctor to sign the discharge paperwork. I was so relieved to have slept through most of my hospital stay.

My fingers were individually wrapped in bulky gauze, which obscured their length. I could tell they were shorter than before the surgery, but I would have to wait to see the results. I was only feeling minimal pain, but I knew from experience it was best not to move or touch them to keep the pain from flaring up.

Instead of feeling nervous about leaving the hospital, I was confident this time that Scott, Dani, and Todd had everything under control. I left secure in the knowledge that I was returning to a peaceful home that would accommodate all of my needs with the most loving care team anyone could imagine. With this surgery behind me, I felt blessed to be slowly regaining control of my life.

CHAPTER 18

HOME FOR THE HOLIDAYS

"Man, when you lose your laugh, you lose your footing."

– Ken Kesey, *One Flew over the Cuckoo's Nest*

Giving Thanks

I intentionally planned my hand surgery for mid-November, knowing Thanksgiving with family would be a welcome distraction from the pain of recovery. Jordan was set to return home with Kai, and Hunter would fly in from Hawaii to join Dani and the rest of our family. Looking forward to having my family home for Thanksgiving made the first days after surgery bearable.

By this point, I had profound recovery fatigue. I was so sick of being sick; I just wanted to be healed. I was on strong painkillers, but the intense pain of having seven fingers amputated kept breaking through between doses. Todd set timers to try to stay on top of it, but just like my leg surgery recovery, the first few days after this surgery were excruciating. I slept as much as I could, trying to get through the toughest part of the recovery.

By the third day post-surgery, we had balanced my medications enough to keep the pain at bay. It helped that I was so excited to have my family home. I was focused on them and didn't want anything to ruin our time together. That mindset had a massive impact on how I committed to overcoming the pain and inconvenience of my surgery. I allowed myself to accept that the week would be different because of my convalescence. Still, I was determined to make the best of it by allowing others to help me and truly appreciating our time together.

Like when I was in the hospital, I felt that the arrival of "guests" made me somehow responsible for them. This was Thanksgiving week, so I reverted to old habits and planned a menu without consulting anyone. I wanted to surprise them by having a plan in place and I ordered an all-inclusive Thanksgiving meal package from an upscale market. I wanted the meal to be perfect.

Just before Jordan arrived, I told Dani about the order.

"We can't have a *store-bought* Thanksgiving," she laughed. "No way. The fun part of Thanksgiving is making a home-cooked meal together!"

"I know, but… I can't do it," I confessed, feeling helpless and disappointed that I was letting my family down when I so wanted to repay all the support they had shown me.

"Mom, we know that. You don't need to," she reassured me. "Hunter, Jordan, Kai, and I will do it. Darrick's coming to help too. We'll all pitch in, and you can help by sharing recipes and cooking tips. It'll be just like the Thanksgiving dinners we've always had. We've got this."

And they did! They nailed it. Hard as it was to step down from my role as head chef, it was equally wonderful to watch my daughters and their future husbands take charge with such grace and ease. We all worked together to create the menu and shopping list, and the kids handled the cooking, with Scott pitching in on the cleaning.

We gave Todd time off the week of Thanksgiving, so he could be with his family while we spent time with ours. This handed my care to Scott and the girls, but they didn't seem to mind at all. Nobody skipped a beat when I needed help getting around in my wheelchair, feeding myself, or using the bathroom. They had become natural caregivers, moving seamlessly between their own tasks and mine.

If there's time during my recovery that most exemplifies the dichotomy of my experience of losing my limbs, it would be that week. There was an unexpected balance: a yin-and-yang of pain and joy, frustration and pleasure, and hopelessness and gratitude.

It ended up being one of the best weeks of my recovery, even though it was also one of the hardest because of both the pain in my fingers and not being able to use my hands. Whenever I felt self-pity or frustration, I looked around at my happy family, and my heart swelled with gratitude for being there to share that time with my loved ones.

What I remember most about that week is the loving care from my family and the wonderful young men who were such an essential part of my daughters' lives and chose to be part of ours as well. They all worked together to make meals, help me with whatever I needed, and support me in my daily routine. They were patient and generous with me. I was thankful to be celebrating Thanksgiving as we always had, grateful for my daughters, and for the two young men who had joined our lives and made our girls so happy.

Just two months prior, my life was nearly taken from me, and I was almost taken from my family. I had survived to host my family in my home once again. That miracle was palpable.

Grateful Birthday to Me

My 53rd birthday was on the Sunday after Thanksgiving. Earlier in the month, in honor of having the privilege of growing older, I set up a fundraiser for Sepsis Alliance. It was my way of saying thank you for all of the information they provided that helped us feel less alone and gave us a roadmap through treatment, recovery, and life beyond sepsis. I set it up on my Facebook Update page and kick-started it with a donation from my family. My friends and extended family, who had been looking for ways to support me in my recovery, made donations that helped raise several thousand dollars. It felt great to spread awareness about sepsis and support the organization that had helped us through the most challenging time of our lives.

On the morning of my birthday, I unexpectedly woke up feeling depressed. The boys had left early that morning, and Jordan would soon be returning to school. Once my birthday was behind me, the celebratory distractions of the week would be gone, and my days would again revolve around recovery from my amputations. The thought of the months of physical therapy and occupational therapy ahead was overwhelming. I had always loved my birthdays, but on that particular one, I felt more grief than excitement. I had a hard time rallying for any type of celebration, unless it was a pity party for one.

I sat up in bed and uncovered my legs, ready for my daily visual reminder that I was still a multiple amputee. When I looked down at my casts, my mood couldn't help but soften. Over the Thanksgiving holiday, I had invited my daughters and nieces to draw on my casts with felt-tip markers. They drew bright, fun pictures with inspirational quotes in vibrant colors. My niece Eliza is a fantastic artist who drew a phoenix rising out of the ashes on one of my legs – a beautiful tribute to my survival and ongoing recovery. On the other leg, my niece Maddy wrote "You are braver than you believe, stronger than you seem, and smarter than you think." That quote from *Winnie the Pooh* and the image of the phoenix were the exact reminders I needed. Despite my doubts, I was going to get through this.

I took a deep breath and reminded myself to stay in the present and keep moving forward, one tiny step at a time. I rang the little pink bell on my bedside table and heard my daughters' excited voices outside my door before they came in and wished me a happy birthday. I put on a smiling face for my family and tried to set aside any sadness.

We had coffee in my favorite spot by our corner windows. The girls and Scott were by my side with fresh fruit and pastries they had prepared as a special breakfast. Cody had come over from Midori's earlier and was seated comfortably on my lap.

Scott gave me a plate of food that I carefully fed myself with my gauze-wrapped fingers, making sure I didn't bump the painful ends on anything as I ate. Cody was extra attentive that morning. He really did have a sixth sense about how I was feeling.

There was a knock on the door, and in walked a man carrying a heavy ceramic pot filled with four huge, white Phalaenopsis orchids. Scott and the girls led him into the living room and showed him a table where he could place this gorgeous display near my morning window. I could feel my sadness fading away, replaced by gratitude. As the florist was leaving, Midori arrived.

"The flowers were Midori's idea," Dani explained. "She knows you've always loved her orchids and thought you needed some of your own."

"She got you this beautiful pot, and Dad will work with the florist to ensure you have blooming orchids year round," added Jordan.

I was deeply touched that everyone had worked together to ensure I would be surrounded by tropical flowers, which would remind me of Hawaii in the drabness of the Seattle winter ahead. With tears in my eyes, I thanked everyone.

"This one is from Dad and us," the girls explained as Midori walked to the kitchen and came back carrying a big gift box with a fancy brand name that I recognized written on the side. "Midori was hiding it at her house."

I knew what it was immediately. Sure enough, I opened the box to find a puffy down jacket in an uplifting shimmery pink color. I had admired it in a store window near my hair salon, but it seemed impractical since I couldn't see myself being out in the cold for more than a few minutes at a time between doctors' appointments. I still struggled to envision any future beyond the life I had.

I was too scared to look ahead, but my family wasn't. They envisioned me in Seattle over the next few months of my recovery and knew I needed beautiful things to remind me of Hawaii and to keep me warm and comfortable during the grey Northwest winter. They suggested I might wear it at a ski resort sometime in the next couple of years. That was a beautiful birthday thought.

Then came a surprise for us all. As we were clearing the dishes, the kitchen door swung open, and my brother-in-law Dan, who lives three hours away in Portland, stepped inside carrying a big, wrapped package. We were delighted by his unplanned arrival. He told us he was "in the area," but I knew that meant he was visiting his lake house an hour-and-a-half away. He'd made a special trip just to deliver this to me. I was so touched.

I opened the package to find a watercolor painting of a hillside scene on an island in Greece that I had visited the year before I fell ill. I recognized it immediately, and memories of that wonderful trip flooded my mind. I had told Dan and his wife, Scott's sister Kristen, how life-changing that trip was for me, and they had remembered.

The painting was even more special because the artist, a friend of Kristen's and Dan's, had experienced a loss similar to mine: she'd had part of her jaw bone removed due to cancer. Kristen had explained that she had a prosthetic cover for her lower face, which she only wore in public to make others feel more comfortable, but she never wore it with her closest family and friends. She told me that her spirit was so much more than her physical body and that she had become entirely comfortable with her new appearance. They were hopeful that I would find comfort in my new life, as she had.

I loved the painting and everything it symbolized. It was a perfect gift!

Looking at the many gifts and loving faces around me, I realized that the smile I had forced for my family's sake had become genuine. I had been happy-crying the entire morning. My pity party had transformed into a love fest, and this was turning out to be a pretty fabulous birthday after all.

On the day I awoke in the ICU two months earlier and saw my black fingertips, it seemed like the worst day of my life. But as I celebrated my birthday, with my amputation surgeries behind me, I decided to reframe that day as one of my best. I was lucky to have survived. I almost didn't get to see Scott again after we parted ways on our separate vacations. I almost didn't get to see my girls after visiting them in California. But I survived my time in the ICU and got a second chance at life.

Instead of just feeling sorry for myself, with my surgeries behind me and living in the body that would take me through the rest of my life, I was appreciative of *getting* to age and being alive to experience a future with my family.

On my 53rd birthday, I came to fully realize a complicated truth: Opposing emotions can coexist. I could feel weak compared to my pre-sepsis fitness *and* be proud of my strengthening body and improving health. I could be sad about the loss of my limbs *and* be happy for my birthday. I was learning to find joy amidst the sadness of my loss.

Fit for the Holidays

By December, I was starting to feel healthier and regaining more strength, both physically and mentally. I continued my PT exercises at home, weaving them into my weekly routine at random times so I wouldn't get sick of them. I liked to mix things up, which isn't surprising as novelty and flexible routines often help people with ADHD to focus. I've always done better exercising on and off throughout the day, using a variety of equipment, rather than sticking to a set workout time and repetitive routines.

I had practiced Pilates and yoga before contracting sepsis, and was eager to get back to them. At the encouragement of a friend, I made an appointment at a Pilates studio with an instructor who had heard my story and was excited to work with me on a program tailored to my new body. I wasn't sure I'd be able to use a reformer (a piece of Pilates equipment that uses springs and body weight for resistance), but my friend assured me the instructor would adapt the exercises to suit my needs. She had adaptive handles and straps designed for people with arthritis, injuries, or disabilities that she planned to use with me.

I felt vulnerable going to her studio, but it was the ideal place because there was never more than one other student and one instructor present at a time. She suggested ways to adapt the standard movements to accommodate my shortened legs, or to use the special hand grips so I could push and pull with only my palms. These sessions not only improved my balance, strength, dexterity, and flexibility, but also helped me become more confident showing my amputations in a safe environment.

What I wanted most to regain was the use of my hands. Trying to get through my days without them working well had been such a challenge. I longed for the day when I could once again pick up an object, turn a doorknob, type on a keyboard, or do any of the myriad things I had once taken for granted. Before that could happen, though, there was one final hurdle to clear.

So Long, Stitches

Two weeks after having my fingers amputated, Todd and I went to the hospital early to grab a donut and a latte at our favorite coffee shop just outside Harborview. Todd always ordered an apple fritter, and I would rotate between a maple bar or an old-fashioned donut. I loved our little morning rituals at the coffee shop before heading into the many appointments we'd been attending over the last few months.

This was a big day because once my stitches were removed from my fingers, I would finally be through my surgical gauntlet. To say that my fingertips had been sore since my surgery would be a huge understatement. The pain was agonizing. The stitches were thick, causing a lot of discomfort at the incision site, and the bulky knot-ends caught on my blankets and dug into my sensitive flesh whenever I touched anything with them, which was often. Old habits are hard to break.

Even after two weeks, my hands kept reaching out and grabbing things before my mind could stop them.

I was scared for that appointment, though, because my fingers were so sore. I couldn't stand the thought of anyone so much as touching them, let alone clipping the stitches from my hypersensitive fingertips. I knew I would have to gather up all my resolve to tolerate the painful and tedious task of cutting the stitches out of all seven of my amputated fingers.

I sat in the waiting room at my hand surgeon's office, wearing my comfy down coat. It was a perfect complement to the soft pink blanket Marnie and Julia had gifted me in the ICU, which I often had on my lap in the wheelchair to hide the space where my legs should have been.

Todd wheeled me into a vacant space in the waiting room next to his chair. Now that I was in a wheelchair, I noticed the empty spaces throughout the waiting areas for wheelchairs or for storing walkers or crutches.

As a new member of the amputee and disability communities, I was starting to become aware of accommodations everywhere I went. I'd noticed accessible parking spaces and bathroom stalls before becoming an amputee, but now I noticed ramps next to stairways, buttons to open doors easily, tables designed for wheelchairs, braille on elevators and ATMs, and verbal cues at crosswalks. I was comforted to realize that the world was becoming increasingly accommodating to people like me.

Todd helped me take off my jacket and tried to fold the fluffy coat into his lap, as if he were rolling up a sleeping bag when breaking camp. It was so full of down, it seemed like a big stuffed animal we carried everywhere we went. Neither of us cared about the added bulk, though. The payoff in comfort was worth the extra effort, and Todd made it clear in everything he did that nothing he helped me with was ever inconvenient.

A familiar nurse called my name in the waiting room. He greeted me like a friend, as many of the hospital staff did, and walked me back to the treatment room to wait for my stitches to be removed.

As I sat with Todd, I was preoccupied with the question of how the surgeon would get scissors between my skin and the stitches to cut them out. In truth, I'd been obsessing about this for weeks. I've always had the frustrating trait of trying to puzzle out in advance how a specialist would solve a problem for which they were specially trained and I had no experience.

One example I think about a lot, which still makes me shudder, is the time I hired a contractor to move a 16-foot sliding glass door from one wall of my house to another to enlarge my living room. When the work crew arrived, they only had two people in their crew, and I couldn't imagine how they would move this colossal piece of glass without dropping or breaking it. It made me so anxious, I couldn't watch; I had to leave the house until they were finished. Of course, it turned out fine, but my stomach still lurches just thinking about it.

As I sat in the treatment room where my stitches would be removed, I was as anxious as I had ever been. All of my relaxation exercises went out the door, and I couldn't stop worrying about how they would cut those tight stitches without hurting my sensitive fingers.

I fidgeted as I waited, using my thumbs to gently touch each of my fingertips, focusing on the tiny gap between the stitches and my skin, and the heightened sensation. Todd tried to distract me by showing me posters featuring diagrams of hands that detailed bones, tendons, and muscles. We looked at each digit carefully and compared it to my fingers, envisioning what was missing. He checked in with me to make sure it wasn't making me feel uncomfortable. It wasn't at all. On the contrary, I found it fascinating.

As I examined my amputated fingers, he reminded me that this was just the beginning of my healing; over the coming months, with lots of occupational therapy and exercises at home, my muscles and tendons would be slowly stretched to improve my range of motion. My hands would eventually begin to move as they had before, without feeling so stiff and sore. I had my doubts about this, but I did my best to take on his positive attitude. I prayed he would be proven right.

A few minutes later, my hand surgeon entered the room with one of his young associates and carefully examined my fingers. I thanked him for saving as much of each of my fingers as he could and for doing such a careful job during the surgery. I could see that he was pleased with the healing process. He assured me that the removal of my stitches would be quick and that the scissors they used were tiny and shouldn't cause me much pain. The younger man with him said he would be the one removing my stitches. He promised he would do it as carefully and quickly as possible. I began to relax.

As promised, he used the tiniest pair of scissors I had ever seen and was as careful as he could be. But I'm not going to lie, it was still an excruciating procedure to endure on seven fingertips. He talked me through the process and allowed me breaks between every stitch.

I was overjoyed that all of my surgeries were entirely behind me. I could now look forward to the next significant milestone in my recovery: getting my prosthetic legs. It felt like an enormous weight had been lifted off me, the one I'd been under ever since I'd seen my dead fingertips in the ICU.

Olive in the House

Now that my fingers were less sensitive, Scott and I agreed it was time to bring our one-year-old puppy, Olive, home from Hawaii. Scott flew alone to Hanalei to close the house up for the winter and to ship both of our dogs to their new homes.

"Bubba" or "Buddy," depending on who you ask, was an elderly hunting dog who wandered into our yard a month after the big Hanalei flood. He was severely malnourished when we found him, or rather, when he found us. We spent weeks nursing him back to health as we searched in vain for his family. He lived outside and slept in the dirt under the shelter of our eaves by our front door, despite having a soft bed and blankets scattered on the covered patio nearby. Once a hunting dog, always a hunting dog.

He was loving and put up with our high-energy puppy, Olive, whom we had adopted a few months before Buddy arrived. They had both been home with me when I got sick, and I like to imagine that Buddy took care of Olive the night she slept outside, as I never woke up to let her in. They had been leading great lives in our absence with a friend who was caretaking our Hanalei house.

Olive would come to our home on Mercer Island, but we had other plans for Buddy. He was elderly and didn't know how to live inside, so it didn't make sense to bring him to the cold and damp of the Pacific Northwest. Hunter, who was living on the Big Island, stepped up and agreed to adopt Buddy, whom he officially renamed "Bubs." Once Scott got Buddy/Bubba/Bubs onto his flight over to Hunter, Scott was able to prepare for his mainland flight home with Olive. Olive was 11months old when I got sick, and still very much "our puppy," so we were anxious to have her back with our family after nearly three months apart.

Now that I was finally "out of the woods" and into my official recovery period, I was excited to have her home, but still worried about her jumping on me and hurting my legs or my hands. Scott assured me she was an older, calmer version of the hyperactive puppy she had been in September, and he was certain she and I would work out a new routine.

When Olive and Scott arrived home, she was skittish about her new surroundings, so Scott kept her outside until I was safely situated on the couch and ready to greet her. He brought her into the living room and kept her on a leash so she couldn't accidentally injure me. Naturally, she was excited to see me, but Scott held her back while she calmed down. When she was calm enough and close enough, I carefully moved my legs off the couch and patted the spot next to me, inviting her to jump up. She cautiously stepped up onto the couch, lay her head in my lap, and rolled over on her back so I could rub her belly. Just like Cody, she seemed to know she needed to be gentle.

Soon, she was licking my face and squirming excitedly. I realized how much I had been missing her love and energy. I was thrilled to have her home again; it was the perfect gift, and a beautiful symbol of my life starting to feel like my own again.

Retail Therapy

Being back in the Seattle area over the holiday season was a treat. I've always loved the seasonal music playing over the store speakers, as well as the Christmas lights strung up in downtown Seattle, Bellevue Square, and University Village – some of my favorite shopping areas. So I was thrilled when Todd suggested we go on a shopping adventure at Bellevue Square. Up to that point, I hadn't been off Mercer Island except to go to appointments at Harborview.

My world was expanding.

In addition to holiday gift shopping, which I was delighted to be able to do, we were on a mission to find me some new clothes: stylish, yet comfy outfits that would fit my new body and make me feel more like the old me, and less like the sick person I had been in the hospital and throughout my recovery.

Driving to the mall, the holiday lights and lavish decorations reminded me of all the years of Christmas shopping I had done there, from college through my young parenting years. I felt like a kid in a candy store returning to this metropolitan mecca of retail shopping after the relatively limited selection in Hawaii.

I was excited *and* nervous, wondering about the logistics of using a wheelchair. *Where would we park? How would I get across the sky bridges into the mall?* I was racking my brain, trying to remember where the elevators were in each department store. I knew we would figure it out when I got there, but my anxious mind wanted to know how it would all work in advance.

Todd had obtained a disability parking placard for me through the Washington State Department of Licensing, so we found parking right up front, near Nordstrom. We parked on the main level, avoiding the skywalks and potential stairways. We crossed the road and found a ramp beside the main stairway that was easily accessible to my wheelchair. When we arrived at the entry door, a bright blue button with a wheelchair symbol was directly in my line of sight. I pressed it with my palm. The doors slowly swung open, revealing another button inside, which opened the next set of doors. It couldn't have gone more smoothly, easing my fears about navigating the mall in a wheelchair.

As Todd pushed me through the store, I noticed other shoppers with various mobility aids, from canes and walkers to crutches and scooters, as well as wheelchairs like mine. This place I thought I knew so well was suddenly a whole new world, one that had always been there alongside my own, just unnoticed by me.

It reminded me of when I was pregnant for the first time. Suddenly, everywhere I looked, I saw other pregnant women and people carrying babies and pushing strollers. I had learned about this phenomenon as a psychology major in college. It's called a frequency illusion: the tendency to notice something more frequently once you've noticed it for the first time. I felt suddenly connected to all these confident people with mobility challenges, and far less alone.

It was uplifting to recognize how many people were out there functioning beautifully in the world with their physical limitations. Our experience at the mall was a success, reassuring me that I, too, could one day confidently navigate the world on my own.

Here Comes Santa Claus

Since 2013, there's been an annual holiday tradition called SUP (Stand-Up Paddleboarding) Santas, where people paddleboard across Lake Washington dressed as Santa Claus, alongside the I-90 floating bridge between Seattle and Mercer Island. It began as a casual activity among friends, but eventually evolved into a community fundraiser for families affected by cancer.

Our house was just half a mile from the bridge, so every year we would sit on our dock, enjoying the seasonal spectacle of festive folks all decked out in red and white, paddling along the floating bridge, waving to cars, and generally making merry. Often, we recognized friends and neighbors among the jolly SUP Santas crew, and Scott had even participated a few times before we moved to Hawaii.

So when a friend reached out and invited Scott to join, I encouraged him to go. I was thankful for this opportunity for him to enjoy a Mercer Island tradition, get out on the water, celebrate the holidays, and spend time with old friends.

I spent the morning with friends and family, listening to holiday music while we watched for the Santas from our house. They were a long way off, but we could see about 30 paddlers dressed in red as Santa Claus, 10 or so dressed in green like Buddy the Elf or the Grinch, plus a handful in assorted holiday pajamas. We cheered as they made their way along the bridge. They were tiny specks when they reached the far side of the bridge, but we watched them loop back toward Mercer Island until we could see their bright costumes again.

We had stepped away from the windows and were starting a Christmas movie when I got a text from Scott that simply said, "Go outside." My friend Melissa, who had come for lunch, wheeled me out to our back deck for a better view of the lake. From the edge of our deck, covered in my warm pink blanket, I saw a group of about 10 SUP Santas near the shore, headed straight toward our house!

Watching them make a beeline for our dock, I realized Scott must have talked them into a side trip to bring me some much-appreciated holiday cheer. I burst into grateful tears as they paddled around our dock, waving and yelling to me, wishing me well, and generally making me feel special and loved.

Seeing Scott among the SUP Santas, looking so happy and carefree after so many months of stress, was a welcome reminder that if we keep seeking it, joy never stops trying to find us. But to receive that joy, we have to slow down and invite it in.

Just Like Old Times

Throughout the holiday season, my family had traditions to keep us busy and bonded. Writing Christmas cards, making Christmas cookies, trimming the tree, and wrapping presents were usually my domain. But not this year. Fortunately, Thanksgiving gave me much-needed practice in letting my family step in and take the reins while I sat back and enjoyed the ride.

While my fingers were healing and we anxiously awaited my first prosthetic legs, we created new traditions as we explored new territory. Dani arranged for us to attend *Enchant Christmas*, which transformed T-Mobile Stadium into a winter wonderland with an ice rink, a variety of festive Christmas trees, tasty treats, and winter holiday activities.

My first thought when Dani told me about it was, *I can't do that. I'm not ready.* She saw the fear in my eyes and explained her plan further.

"Don't worry. I called ahead and asked, and they have wheelchair access. I know where to get in. Dad will drop us off at the main entrance and there's someone at the gate who will let us cut in front of the line in the wheelchair. Dad will park the car nearby in accessible parking so it's easy for us to leave when you're ready to go, and he'll meet us inside. I know where to meet him." My daughter knew me well enough to know I needed to walk through each step of the process mentally beforehand, or I would be gripped with anxiety until we arrived.

Going to that event was significant on two levels: not only was it a treasured holiday memory with my family, replacing the outdoor light show we traditionally attended at a local nursery, but it was proof that, with a bit of planning, a lot of the possibilities I'd dismissed were back on the table.

With the success of the *Enchant Christmas* show under my belt, I felt confident enough to attend *Snowflake Lane*, the holiday parade at Bellevue Square we'd attended every year when we lived there a decade ago. We often knew people who performed in it, either as drum corps members, or dancers, so it had become one of our favorite family Christmas traditions.

The girls and I went with my nephew Darrick while Scott was out of town for a couple of days. Darrick had been on this journey with us since my first week awake in the hospital, so I knew I was in good hands with the girls and him leading the way. We parked at the mall and made our way out to the main parade route.

The girls walked ahead, and Darrick wheeled me through the crowd, navigating around groups of people to get to a place where I could see the snowflake lights, parade floats, and drummers. As we watched the parade, one of the performers walked right in front of my wheelchair on impossibly tall stilts, navigating the tight crowd as though it were the easiest thing in the world. His legs must have been five feet tall. I looked up to see his face in full clown makeup and realized: *he's just a kid!*

I turned back to Darrick and called out over the noise of the parade, "If that young boy can walk on stilts, I can figure out how to walk on prosthetic legs!"

We shared an enthusiastic high five as my doubts evaporated, "Yeah, you can!"

And for the first time since realizing I would lose my lower legs, I believed I could.

All I Want for Christmas

Throughout December, despite the welcome distraction of the holidays, I couldn't get my mind off the exciting possibility that I would get my first prosthetic legs before Christmas. This was based on the estimate from my surgeon that I would need to heal for 10 weeks after my amputation surgery. Christmas Eve was just under 10 weeks from my surgery. I set that as my aspirational goal.

Despite our best efforts and my speedy healing, we learned a few days before Christmas that my appointment to fit the legs wouldn't be until my prosthetist Stephanie's return from her holiday break on

December 27th. I was disappointed, but the activities surrounding Christmas helped me find the patience to wait just a few days longer.

Looking back, I realize that the holiday season of 2018 was a turning point in my recovery. My perspective began to shift from one of loss to one of gratitude, which really blossomed on my first Christmas as an amputee. It would have been exciting to have my new legs, but I realized I'd already received the greatest gift I could wish for: a beautiful Christmas full of love and gratitude, surrounded by my family.

CHAPTER 19

TWO STEPS FORWARD, ONE STEP BACK

"The Journey of 1000 miles begins with a single step."

– Lao Tzu

One Step Forward

December 27, 2018

I woke up that morning giddy with anticipation.

Today's the day I get my new legs and feet!

Scott helped me get ready while Todd made us breakfast. We listened to upbeat music in honor of the occasion. Lady Gaga's "Shallow" and David Guetta's "Titanium" played on repeat.

Scott helped me get dressed, then brushed my thinning hair as I watched him in the full-length mirror. My eyes were drawn to the empty space below my residual limbs where my feet used to be. My heart ached, as it always did when I saw my truncated legs with no feet. Even writing this, my chest contracts viscerally.

I usually avoided looking at my legs at all. It was a painful shock every time. The mirror upstairs in the bathroom where I showered remained covered with a towel for months, because seeing the space where my feet should have been made my heart heavy. That glaring emptiness was the unwelcome reminder that this long nightmare was, in fact, real.

But knowing that in just a few hours I would try on my new prostheses, bringing an end to the long weeks I'd spent without lower legs, made me want to take in the full effect one last time. It wasn't easy. I was still hesitant to look at that part of my body I'd been avoiding for so long.

Watching Scott brush my hair reminded me of how hard the past few months had been. I had never felt so helpless. I was reliant on everyone else to care for me. At the same time, I was overwhelmed with gratitude for how well my friends and family had nurtured and protected me.

Will that change when I have my new legs? I hope so.

I was becoming more capable every day. Dani had recently left to be with Hunter for New Year's before heading to San Diego to return to work, and Jordan was leaving for her semester in Rome in a few days. I could feel my family handing the reins of my life back to me. It was bittersweet.

My eyes shifted from the safety of my loving husband to my thinning hair, looking stringy and sparse. I could tell he didn't know how to style it to make it look thicker, but it melted my heart watching him try. It reminded me of watching him care for our girls when they were younger. He had such love and compassion in his eyes.

I looked at my makeup and noticed the glow in my cheeks, the sparkle in my eyes, and the way I filled out the clothes that had hung on my weak frame two months prior. I sat strong and tall in my chair, wearing the puffer jacket I got for my birthday, which felt like a warm hug from my entire family.

I allowed my eyes to drop lower. I was wearing baggy sweatpants hanging empty past my calves, waiting for the new legs I would be getting that day. I could never decide whether to let my pants hang or tuck the ends under my thighs. It didn't really matter, though; nothing could hide my disfigurement.

Security Blankets

As I had done every day since my amputations, I would put a favorite blanket on my lap like an invisibility cloak to protect my lower legs from prying eyes. I wasn't comfortable showing this part of myself in public.

I had bestowed on these blankets the power that my bed sheets used to have when I was a little girl: the power to protect me from the scariest monsters. Blankets were my shields.

Tiffany had wrapped me in a blanket from my home in Hanalei on that first day in the hospital. It was on our bed, a cozy nest for Olive, who slept with us every night. It made me feel safe on the frantic ride to the hospital and through the early days of my sepsis journey. That blanket accompanied me to Queen's Medical Center on Oahu. It protected me through my time in the ICU, until Marnie and Julia upgraded it to a softer, more luxurious one. Since then, I'd been given several other blankets that concealed my missing feet and comforted me wherever I went, including one handmade by a friend from church who prayed for me as she made it. I was never without a blanket.

After my amputations, I felt comfortable sitting on the couch among family without my legs. When anyone else was around, I would grab the nearest blanket, throw it over my legs, and bunch it up at the bottom to create the illusion of feet. My fingers were easier to disguise: just by curling them, I could hide them in my palms.

I often felt silly putting that effort in when friends were visiting. They knew I lost my lower legs. But that morning, as I sat in my wheelchair looking in the mirror at the space where my feet should be, I realized I wasn't doing it for them. I was doing it for *me*.

I was the one who didn't want to see my legs without their feet, or to be seen without them.

Will I still need a security blanket after today?

Mirror, Mirror

Looking in that mirror, I pictured myself as I used to be, standing strong, my feet planted firmly on the Earth. Tears welled up in my eyes as memories of my prior life floated away like wispy tendrils of smoke.

That's not me anymore. I am now, and will forever be, a bilateral below-knee amputee who is missing partial fingers on both hands. I will be using prosthetic legs for the rest of my life.

A tear rolled off my lower lashes and down my cheek. Scott put his hand on my shoulder, reminding me that I wasn't alone. Our sad eyes met in the mirror as his brows furrowed. I could tell how helpless he felt. This was one of the rare occasions when he let me see that this journey was impacting him nearly as much as it was impacting me. I knew that if he could trade places with me and take away all my pain, he would do it in a heartbeat. I felt the strength of knowing we were in this together.

I wiped away my tears, put my hand on his, and told him I was ready. As we left the house to head to the hospital, I felt like I was leaving my recovery behind me and heading toward my future.

With my new lower legs and feet, I could begin the journey toward independence as I learned to walk. There would no longer be an empty space at the bottom of my legs when I sat in my wheelchair. Children wouldn't cower behind their parents when they noticed my footless body passing them in public. I would be able to put a foot on the floor and pivot onto a chair or couch, rather than performing a complicated gymnastics routine every time I transferred from my wheelchair.

I would feel connected to the planet once again.

Without my feet, I felt like I was floating in space, untethered, as if I would drift away without my friends and family connecting me to the Earth. Before I became sick, I would walk barefoot or sit on the grass to ground myself and meditate, sensing the energy of that connection. I longed for that feeling again.

With my new legs, I would be able to look down and see toes poking out of my jeans. I would see my new feet, size seven, as they had always been, touching the floor where my old feet used to be.

"My new feet," I rehearsed silently, *"My feet."*

Daring to Dream

With Todd pushing my wheelchair, we followed my prosthetist, Stephanie, to the exam room. Scott and Todd helped me onto the chair-height examination table, where Stephanie had fitted my sockets during my prior appointment. Todd sat nearby, ready to assist me if needed, while Scott took videos to document this monumental day.

The energy in our group was palpable. I could tell that even Stephanie was excited about this visit. It must feel amazing for a prosthetist to deliver new limbs to a person who has lost their own.

Stephanie and I had chosen my feet based on my expected activity level, which she had determined a few weeks earlier during an interview about my past activities and future aspirations.

I felt so hopeless at the time, I didn't dare dream about what I might be able to do in the future. I was too stuck in the painful present. I downplayed my desires, telling Stephanie I just wanted to be able to do basic things unassisted, like showering and getting dressed, walking around my house, and cooking.

"One day," I said softly, afraid I was dreaming too big, "I would like to climb the stairs to my bedroom on my own."

Scott was stunned that this was the best I could do when dreaming of my future. I glowed with gratitude as he took over and proudly told her all the activities I had enjoyed before my amputations. He shared with her our dreams for my future.

"She wants her life back. She fishes on rivers and in the ocean. She hikes, wakeboards, snowboards, rides bikes, drives a car, and travels the world. She was a gymnast for years when she was younger. She played volleyball and soccer in high school. She's not afraid to tackle tasks like fixing a toilet, changing a faucet, climbing a ladder to clean windows, caulking cracks, and painting walls. She became a certified yoga teacher when we moved to Hawaii and completed her first 5K run two years ago."

Scott's faith sparked my confidence, daring me to dream about all that could be possible. With him supporting and encouraging me, I started to imagine living a life similar to the one I had before becoming an amputee.

"Actually," I chimed in, "I would love to watercolor paint again, go snorkeling, and maybe even scuba dive. And one day, I want to be able to babysit and play with my grandkids."

With a warm smile, Stephanie responded, "I'll do all I can to help you do all of those things."

She encouraged me to make an appointment with a recreational therapist who could help me become more active within my current abilities and continue working with me as I began walking. Todd made that appointment for me as soon as we got home.

Stephanie reassured me that, given my fitness level, I might eventually be able to perform a variety of activities, such as running, swimming, riding a bike, and navigating uneven terrain. I was thrilled to discover that I qualified for the highest level of athletic prostheses! Despite all I had been through, I could still lead an active life.

My heart fluttered as I imagined this possibility. But doubt snuck back in.

Am I setting my sights too high? I'm missing both my lower legs in my 50's. Am I too old for such a strong recovery? I don't think I can handle any more loss or disappointment.

Even as I sat on the examination table watching Stephanie assemble my new legs, the most I could allow myself to imagine was seeing myself in the mirror, in my wheelchair, with legs where my residual limbs had been that morning. I was still so afraid that I wouldn't be able to walk and would need a wheelchair for the rest of my life, even with prosthetic legs.

The Moment We'd Been Waiting For

Stephanie brought my legs over and presented them like newborn twins, taking the time to point out every detail. She showed me that each leg consisted of several components, listing names I didn't yet understand but would soon become a part of my regular vocabulary.

She laid out a plethora of boxes on the padded table where I sat, opened each one, and explained the contents. Scott, Todd, and I were rapt. We had been waiting for this moment for months and didn't want to miss a thing.

There were many parts to these new legs of mine. Before seeing all the boxes and components, I had thought I could just slip them on and go. It was more complicated than I'd anticipated. I could tell that no matter how much my medical team educated me, I wouldn't feel comfortable leaving the hospital and managing them on my own. I was relieved that Scott and Todd were there to learn with me and would help me when we returned home.

The hollow sockets were designed to fit over my residual limbs. I had come into her office a couple of weeks earlier, and Stephanie had made casts of both my lower legs so the prostheses would fit me perfectly. The material was about 1/8 inch thick and appeared to be some type of laminated fiberglass.

My sockets were custom laminated with a decorative, swirly, ocean-blue fabric. Visiting fabric shops a few weeks earlier with my daughters and nieces had been exciting, as I was looking for the perfect material to adorn my first prosthetic legs. It was empowering to get to express my own personal style. I couldn't wait to finally wear them.

When I was still in the hospital in Hawaii, I had made the decision *not* to hide my prosthetic sockets and their metal components under silicone shells that resembled natural skin. A big part of my identity had always been my authenticity, and I didn't want my amputations to change that. Living in Hawaii, wearing shorts most days, they would be visible for all to see. If I had to be an amputee, I was going to ***rep*** being an amputee, with swirly blue sockets, metal ankles, and all.

My Muses

I was inspired by Amy Purdy and Lauren Wasser, both bilateral amputees, whom my daughters had discovered online before I had my amputations. Amy is a Paralympic snowboarding champion, a finalist on "Dancing with the Stars," and an acclaimed international speaker. Lauren is a wildly successful international fashion model and talented basketball player. Both women proudly display their sockets and the metal components of their lower legs in public appearances and photo shoots. Their confidence is infectious.

Dani and Jordan showed me photos of Amy all over the internet wearing beautiful gowns and receiving well-deserved awards. On the red carpet, she wears black carbon-fiber legs and cute high-heeled sandals with adjustable prosthetic feet. In her snowboarding photos, she wears her snow pants rolled up to her knees, showcasing her high-tech custom snowboarding legs and feet.

Lauren also proudly features her legs in haute couture ads for top designers. She's known as "The Girl with the Golden Legs" for her signature gold prostheses, often paired with matching gold basketball shoes.

Before we found Amy and Lauren, I was planning to hide my legs with skin-like covers and wide-leg pants. But once we saw these two powerful women, we began referring to my future prostheses as my "sexy cyborg legs," putting a positive spin on the misfortune of my limb loss.

Our use of the word "cyborg" was pretty tongue-in-cheek at the time. Still, upon investigation, I discovered that a cyborg is a living organism with restored or enhanced abilities resulting from artificial components, which does apply to my use of prosthetic limbs. I don't identify as a cyborg today, but I could if I wanted to!

My "Barbie Feet"

Stephanie described all the components of my prostheses as she assembled them. Metal posts, or "pylons," extended from the bottom of my sockets to mechanical metal feet, with a pivoting mechanism that allowed them to mimic ankle motion. I had never seen feet like these before – all the prostheses I had seen had molded-plastic feet that looked natural. To my relief, Stephanie covered the mechanical-looking metal feet with a tear-resistant Kevlar sock and the Barbie-like foot shells I had been expecting. My new feet had a split next to the big toe, which would allow me to wear sandals, just as I had always done in Hawaii.

There were silicone sock-like sleeves to pad and protect my residual limbs, and larger silicone suspension sleeves to connect the tops of my sockets to my thighs and hold my legs in place.

Now that everything was laid out on the table, it was time for me to don my new legs. I pulled my sweatpants up to my thighs and put on each silicone liner, rolling them up my lower legs and knees like socks. While I did that, Stephanie slid the large black silicone suspension sleeves onto the top of my prosthetic legs, and rolled them down slightly so I could fit my legs inside. When she finished attaching them, she set my new legs on the floor in front of me.

"Give them a try," she encouraged.

I sat at the edge of the table, dangling my legs off the side, and tried to slide my legs into the sockets for the first time. It was harder than I expected. I was worried my legs didn't fit the sockets, and I wouldn't be able to try walking in them or take them home that day.

"Don't worry, I can make adjustments to make them fit," she promised, calming my concerns.

Stephanie explained that my calves were "still a bit bulbous," meaning my lower legs were slightly larger than the openings of the prostheses. The openings couldn't be changed too much because they had to support my knees for the sockets to hold my weight properly. She reassured me that it would get easier to fit them into the sockets in the future. This was pretty common and wouldn't be a problem for long because my legs would shrink over time as they lost muscle and fluids while healing from the amputations.

As it turned out, with a bit of shimmying back and forth and Stephanie's help applying downward pressure, my legs fit into the sockets like a glove. She showed me how to roll up both suspension sleeves so they gripped my thighs, keeping my sockets securely in place. They felt snug but comfortable.

While sitting on the table, I leaned over my knees to look down at my feet. Stephanie had put ankle socks and my old tennis shoes over my feet, so from my angle, they looked exactly the same as they had before. It was thrilling to feel like I had feet again!

I was immediately uplifted, feeling my feet firmly planted on the ground. I lifted each leg and set it down solidly. I was once again connected to the Earth. Tears filled my eyes. I could already feel my life changing.

Two Steps Forward

Stephanie rolled a walker in front of me, reached out her hand, and said, "Do you want to stand up?"

I was scared, but found confidence when I looked into the huge smiles on Scott's and Todd's faces. Todd took my arm, and Scott filmed a video of me for the girls and my parents as I held onto the walker in front of me. My prostheses were so stiff at the ankles that I couldn't get myself up from the table on my first attempt.

Stephanie showed me how to slide my feet back a bit so my knees were ahead of them, and I hoisted myself into a standing position for the first time since I'd been hospitalized with sepsis. I was afraid it would hurt, so I put most of my weight in my arms. I wobbled as I tried to balance, but Todd supported me while Scott cheered me on and captured it all on video.

I felt so empowered standing on my own two feet again!

Looking over at Todd, I realized he had never seen me stand. I gave him a huge hug as he helped me balance, celebrating my first time standing on prosthetic legs.

My eyes met Scott's, and we smiled at one another, acknowledging that this moment was washing away the doubts and fears we had felt earlier that morning.

I was surprised it didn't hurt more. I had been worried that the weight of my body would press down on the tender area at the bottom of my residual limbs, where they had been amputated. But that wasn't how it felt at all. Much of my weight was being held in the upper portion of my sockets on the sides of my knees and in my calves, with a minimum amount of pressure on my surgical scars and fragile amputated limbs. I felt a lot of pressure in my lower legs, but it didn't hurt.

With Stephanie's encouragement, I leaned less on the walker and began putting more weight on my legs, taking a few tiny steps forward so she could see how my legs balanced my weight. I told her I felt a couple of tight spots on my lower legs, so she had me sit back down on the examination table while she took them away and adjusted them.

When she returned, I used the metal walker for my first real walk as an amputee. With Stephanie by my side, I slowly walked from her office, crossed the hall, and went into the physical therapy room, where I was met with my wheelchair so I could take a break.

After I had rested and celebrated my first big walk, Stephanie invited me to stand between two parallel bars and slowly walk down a short walkway to get a feel for my new legs. The bars helped me improve my balance and posture, which were both crucial for walking independently. I was euphoric to be doing it with minimal support on my first try!

I was afraid I might be dreaming, or might not be able to balance without the bars, but my doubts were quickly replaced by elation as I saw myself in the mirror, *walking*. Picture me with the joyous yet apprehensive face of a toddler taking their first steps. Scott, Todd, and Stephanie were beaming with pride. Their love and confidence buoyed me.

If you want to see how it feels to walk on prosthetics for the first time, look up the viral online video, "Look Maggie! I'm walking." Nobody has ever expressed this joy better than that sweet, precious boy.

You're welcome.

Patience, Patience, Patience

When our appointment ended, Stephanie emphasized that I should use a walker at home and shouldn't attempt to walk without it until I had strengthened my legs and improved my balance. She taught me one of the most important lessons of recovery from amputations: injury would mean a longer recovery. I would risk causing damage to my fragile residual limbs that could result in further surgery, and even make it impossible to walk.

To protect my new legs, she gave me a schedule for how long I should wear them each day, starting with standing for less than a couple of minutes and taking only a few steps at a time. She cautioned that I would progress slowly as my prostheses became more comfortable, and would eventually graduate from a walker to a cane until I felt secure walking on my own.

She asked me to take it easy and pace myself, as even a small blister on one of my residual limbs could force me out of my prostheses until it was fully healed. To reach my goal to walk again, I needed to prioritize avoiding injury. That included slips and falls as well as more minor injuries like ingrown hairs, blisters, or abrasions on my residual limbs that would prevent me from wearing them.

I would continue seeing Stephanie every couple of weeks and a physical therapist twice a week for a few weeks, then gradually reduce my visits as I gained strength, confidence, and balance. I was reassured that I could always get emergency appointments if I needed adjustments to my prostheses.

Feeling Grounded

When we got home, Jordan was packing to leave for her semester abroad in Italy. One of my greatest joys during that holiday season was being able to stand up from my wheelchair that day to hug my daughter and tell her how proud and grateful I was for her support while she stayed in school. I was so happy she got to see me stand before she left for Rome.

My friends and family had all been through so much, supporting me through the unknowns of my recovery. I couldn't wait to go on my Facebook update page and announce to the world that I now had legs and was learning to walk. So many demons were put to rest that day for all of us who worried I might never walk again.

New Year's Revolution

December 31, 2018, was the end of the most challenging year I had ever experienced. In the last three months, I had gone from a healthy, fit woman to one who nearly lost her life and was now living as a multiple amputee who required assistance for mobility.

My heart still ached because of all the loss I had experienced, but my prosthetic legs represented new hope, along with the promise of a brighter future where my health and fitness could return, and I could reclaim a life more like the one I nearly lost. I was ready to move forward, confident I would have smooth sailing ahead. My New Year's resolution that year was to walk unassisted by spring.

A Star is Born

When I was 12, my mom and I shared a special bond over the movie *A Star is Born*. She had loved the 1951 version starring Kathleen Crowley and could hardly wait to see the remake starring her favorite singer, Barbra Streisand. I remember her excitement in sharing the movie with me. She cautioned me that the story was sad, but she knew that Barbra Streisand's singing would be captivating. We loved the music so much that we played the album nonstop. It was the soundtrack to that year of my life and I still know all the words by heart.

In the summer of 2018, before I fell ill with sepsis, I saw the trailer for a new remake of the film starring Lady Gaga, an incredibly talented singer. I remember getting goosebumps and having tears well up as I heard a clip from the song "Shallow," a power ballad that touches your soul. If you've seen the trailer or the movie, you know what I mean. I couldn't wait to see it with my girls.

"Shallow," along with several other songs from the album, was playing in my hospital room throughout my recovery. The lyrics, "I'm off the deep end, watch as I dive in; I'll never meet the ground," held a strong, personal meaning for me, independent of what the lyrics were intended to represent.

I'd never been in a more difficult situation in my life. At the beginning, I felt like I was in way over my head, and might drown before ever reaching solid ground again. The words echoed my pain and fears and helped me break through to my sorrow, allowing me to grieve my loss. But at the same time, that powerful music and Lady Gaga's passion seemed to be promising redemption.

That song had come to mean everything to me. It was the embodiment of ambivalence: opposing feelings coexisting. I could feel like I was drowning *and* believe I would break free and find solid footing again. Both could be true simultaneously.

The movie was scheduled for release while I was at Queen's in Hawaii. I cried when I realized I wouldn't be able to see it as early as I had planned. It became one more thing I had lost to sepsis. But my family assured me I would see it in a theater. They promised to take me when I got out of the hospital, reassuring me that movie theaters had wheelchair-accessible spaces.

As promised, to celebrate getting my new legs, Scott and Dani arranged for me to see *A Star is Born* in a theater near our home. They offered to buy wheelchair tickets, but I was unsure what the reserved spaces would be like and worried about where Dani and Scott would sit. We weren't sure whether to buy three wheelchair seats or if there was a different way to get tickets for the people who would accompany me. It was frustrating not knowing how to navigate the world in my new body. I was afraid to try accessible seats and insisted that we buy regular seats that were close to the main aisle, and we could figure it out when we got there.

When we arrived at the theater, we paid close attention as we passed the accessible seats and noticed the open spaces reserved for wheelchair users, with regular seats adjacent to them. I made a note to try that next time.

Thanks to my new legs, I was able to walk the three or four steps to my seat. I was uncomfortable wearing my legs throughout the movie, but I felt self-conscious about removing them, so I spent a lot of time shuffling around in my seat, trying to get comfortable. Eventually, I slipped off my legs and laid my coat across my lap and lower legs to feel less conspicuous. At the end of the movie, I slipped my legs back on before the lights came back on and used the seats for balance, as I walked the few steps to my wheelchair without a hitch.

It wasn't a perfect experience, but it was a glimpse into my future, where things like going to the movies were back on the menu for me.

I'd tried something scary and was rewarded with hope that I might regain more of what I thought had been taken from me by sepsis and my amputations.

With a glimpse into the dynamic life I could still lead as an amputee, I felt empowered as I left the theater that night. "Shallow" remains one of my favorite songs and is a reminder that even when it seems like I'm in over my head, solid ground might be ahead if I just keep swimming.

The Write Stuff

"I can't even write my name," I lamented to my friend over lunch one day.

Though I'd been doing puzzles and occupational therapy to try to regain dexterity in my hands, the truth is that the loss of my legs and relearning how to walk with prosthetics had almost completely overshadowed the loss of my fingers.

Melissa, an Occupational Therapist by training, took my statement as a challenge.

"Show me," she instructed, handing me a piece of paper and a pencil with a foam tube around it. The tube, which resembled a tiny pool noodle, made it easier for me to grip small objects, such as writing instruments and cutlery.

To my shock and our mutual delight, we discovered that, with the help of the foam tube, I could write my name shakily, but legibly.

"Here, try these," she suggested next, handing me a pair of chopsticks.

I laughed and shook my head, "There's no way I can use those!"

"Just try," she insisted, showing me how to rest one chopstick in the crook between my thumb and pointer finger, and use the end of my shortened pointer finger to lever the other one up and down.

To my even greater shock, I realized she was right: using chopsticks was easy for me, maybe even easier than using a fork. To celebrate this discovery, I ate the rest of my salad with chopsticks.

That experience made me wonder what else might be easier for me than I'd imagined. Chopping vegetables? Typing? Cutting my own food? I spent the rest of that day experimenting and quickly discovered that, while some things were still challenging, all were possible with a bit of accommodation plus ingenuity and patience. Based on my experience, I knew that with practice, all of these new skills would get easier over time.

A New Symbol of Our Love

As I began to get my life back in order, I grew increasingly frustrated that my wedding ring still couldn't fit over the swollen knuckle on my ring finger, and likely never would again. Even if I got a bigger size, I realized I would feel self-conscious calling attention to my hand, which now had four partially amputated fingers.

Scott suggested we replace it with something more comfortable for me. I wanted it to be meaningful and symbolic of our marriage, while also representing this time in our lives. We decided on a fancy watch.

Together, we designed the perfect wedding watch for me. I chose a platinum band, since my wedding ring had been platinum, with rose gold in the middle to symbolize the pink bracelets my family and friends had worn to honor my recovery. I selected a mother-of-pearl face to symbolize the beauty of Hawaii and its oceans, with little diamonds marking five-minute increments around the face of the clock to represent my friends and family who surrounded me during the hardest time of my life.

The watch itself symbolized every minute Scott had been watching over me during my illness. He barely left my side, and if he was gone for any significant length of time, he always arranged for one of my children, Todd, or another trusted friend or close relative to be there for me. It was the perfect new symbol of our marriage and life together, encompassing not just us, but also our family and community.

Upward and Onward

When I told my friend Amy that Scott still had to carry me up to bed, she encouraged me to try to get myself up the stairs on my own. I hadn't really thought about trying until she suggested it. I was worried about injuring the end of my lower legs, which were still sensitive from the amputations and further irritated by my new prostheses.

She reminded me that my back, core, and arms were plenty strong and suggested I try pulling myself up backwards, one step at a time, without the use of my legs. She demonstrated it first, then encouraged me to try it while she kept an eye on me so I wouldn't fall down the stairs or injure my lower legs. After my success with writing and using chopsticks, I felt confident enough to give it a try.

I lowered myself out of my wheelchair onto the floor and scooted over to the stairs until my back was up against the first step. I leaned back, put both of my palms on the edge of the step above me, and pulled my bottom up onto the first stair. Just like writing my name, it was easier than I had imagined. I didn't need to push with my legs at all and could hold them up as I scooted my body farther up the stairs.

With Amy in front of me, I practiced reversing these motions and lowered myself down the stairs one step at a time. It worked like a charm. I could now go upstairs and downstairs on my own if I wanted or needed to. We could keep my wheelchair on the main floor and put the wheelchair we borrowed from a friend upstairs for me to use while I was on the second floor. This gave me a great sense of security and accomplishment, and got me one step closer to navigating my world independently.

That success inspired me to try to get out of the house on my own in case of an emergency. Amy helped me practice crawling across the floor, pulling the door open, and scooting myself out onto the porch and down the steps to my patio, where I could safely wait for help. Again, I felt proud of my progress, secure in the knowledge that I could navigate my home without my legs, as needed. These lessons still provide me comfort, knowing I can move around in an emergency if I can't reach my legs.

One Step Back

Okay, Aphrodite, please make me feel beautiful again.

This is what I thought as the stunning stylist at Gene Juarez, appropriately named after the Greek Goddess of love and beauty, gently ran her fingers through what was left of my hair.

After my surgeries were behind me, I began to admit to myself that I was losing hair. I noticed it every time I brushed it or showered, but I had been in denial that it was becoming a significant issue. I started stretching out the time between washings, hoping it would slow the loss, and pulled it back into a little ponytail to try to hide how thin it had become. I think I believed that if nobody else said I was losing my hair, I wouldn't ever have to face it. Eventually, though, it was impossible to camouflage, even from myself.

I was surprised by the depth of the grief I felt as larger and larger wads of hair fell out in the shower or stayed in my hairbrush. I've joked that it was almost harder to lose my hair than my legs. This is an exaggeration, of course, but it hit me hard because it happened on the home stretch of my recovery – the last mile of the marathon I had been running for nearly four months. I just didn't feel like I had the strength left to deal with even one more loss.

I felt my recovery slipping backwards, and I couldn't handle it. Just as I was getting back on my feet, gaining strength, and feeling in control of my life again, the loss of my hair made me look sick and weak. My newfound confidence crumbled into depression and defeat.

I judged myself harshly for my grief, labeling it as "vanity," rather than showing myself the same compassion I would show any woman going through that kind of physical loss. Todd and Scott were worried about me and suggested we talk with my doctor to see what she would recommend. I'm not sure if they scheduled the appointment to talk about my hair or to adjust my antidepressants, but I'm grateful that they stepped in when they could see I was overwhelmed.

I learned that Telogen Effluvium, rapid hair loss from physical or emotional shock, is quite common after significant trauma. It didn't make losing my beloved hair any easier to accept, but it did make me feel a little less alone. I was frustrated that my medical team hadn't mentioned the possibility of hair loss to me, but I found out later that my family knew about it. It doesn't happen to everyone, so they just didn't want to add to my worries.

I was given no guarantees about when my hair loss would stop, but my doctor saw new short hairs coming in all over my head, which was encouraging. She was confident that my hair would regrow. She suggested that it might be easier to grow out and accept if I cut my hair short.

Although I had been successfully fooling myself that my hair looked fine and I didn't need to cut it, when I got home and looked in the mirror, I felt like blinders had been removed from my eyes. My hair was no more than an airy fringe; I could see through the strands that stretched down below my shoulders like a sheer curtain. I took as much control of the situation as I could, deciding it was time to let go of the long hair I had sported while living in Hawaii and embrace an edgier haircut to go with the new me.

Dani scheduled an appointment to have my hair cut and styled, hoping it would make me feel refreshed and more like my old self. Before the appointments, she and Jordan sent me dozens of texts with photos of celebrities and models with cute short haircuts. Scott comforted me by reminding me that I had sported short hair when I was younger and it looked great. I chose a pixie cut similar to a style I wore after my girls were born.

As Dani pushed my wheelchair into the salon, I felt vulnerable about cutting off my long hair and anxious about all the people who would be there. The salon was far more public than a dark movie theater or a restaurant where I could hide my legs under a table. I felt like I would be very conspicuous in my wheelchair, getting most of my hair chopped off. To ease me into the experience, Dani parked me in the waiting room and checked me in so I didn't need to talk with anybody until the stylist came to get me.

"Hi, I'm Aphrodite," she said with a warm smile, "I'll be taking care of you today." Her name, which reminded me of my trip to Greece, was a good omen that I had come to the right place.

I felt the need to explain to her why I was in a wheelchair. I gave her a quick summary of what had happened to me, and she nodded with compassion. Clearly, she had seen a lot of people in wheelchairs in the salon, so she didn't make a big deal about it. It was refreshing to realize I wasn't alone.

Dani stood protectively nearby as I got my hair done. I avoided making eye contact with any of the other patrons, looking only at Dani, Aphrodite, and myself in the mirror.

So you can imagine how startled I was when the woman next to me leaned over and said, "Excuse me?"

Oh no. What's she going to ask me?

Feeling suddenly self-conscious, I looked at her face to see if I recognized her. I didn't. Dani protectively swooped in to join the conversation.

"Are you a friend of Amy Green's?" the woman asked.

I was. Amy was a dear friend who had been encouraging me throughout my recovery.

The woman explained that she knew my story through Amy and had been praying for me since she heard I was in the ICU. I was embarrassed to realize I was starting to cry; it was overwhelmingly touching to know that strangers like this kind woman had been praying for my family and me. Dani comforted me by gently cradling my shoulder.

"I'm so happy my prayers were answered," the woman beamed. "You survived! I can't imagine what you've been through. I hope you know how strong and brave you are."

To be seen with such compassion was powerful. This was the first time it began to sink in that my story, and all that my family and I were going through, was meaningful to people even beyond my immediate circle of friends.

Aphrodite waited patiently for our conversation to end before showing me how to use mousse and a blow-drier to make my hair look thicker than it was. An immediate sense of renewal washed over me as I took in my reflection with this fun new look. In that mirror, I saw myself as a brave and beautiful woman, ready to step into her new life.

CHAPTER 20

WHEN IN ROME

"Life begins at the end of your comfort zone."

– Neale Donald Walsch

An Unexpected Journey

"There's something we haven't told you," Midori announced one morning over breakfast.

I looked over at Scott, who squeezed my hand, smiling reassuringly.

"Well," Midori continued, "you know I'm still planning to visit Jordan in Rome."

I knew. Before all this happened, we had planned a girls' trip to Rome during Jordan's semester studying abroad, something all three of us had been looking forward to. Though I was sad to miss out because I was still recovering, I took comfort in knowing Midori would still be going, even if I couldn't.

It had been heart-wrenching for Jordan to leave while I was still healing, but it was important to all of us that she continue on her path and not allow this tragedy to knock her off of it. I knew how much she was looking forward to seeing Midori and reconnecting with everything that was happening at home.

Midori went on to excitedly explain that she, Dani, Jordan, and Scott had secretly set a goal for me to be able to accompany Midori to Rome in a wheelchair by April. They knew I was initially too overwhelmed to hope for such a possibility, so they had waited to announce their plan until now, when I was starting to get comfortable walking on my prosthetic legs.

"We all think you'll be able to do it with no problem, if you're willing to try," Midori reassured, presenting me with a lavender Lululemon backpack she'd bought me for the occasion. It had plenty of pockets to hold everything I would need to keep handy for the trip.

I was overjoyed for a moment, but then a flood of worries rushed in as my brain flipped through all the horrible things that could go wrong. *How am I going to fly for 14 hours on an airplane and spend a week in Rome, when I can barely handle a trip to the movies?* I presented all the obstacles I could think of, but they were way ahead of me and had a solution for each one.

Because I would be flying with prosthetic legs for the first time, Scott had booked me in first class so I could sleep in a lie-flat seat and wouldn't have to walk far to use the restroom. He also bought and installed special wheels with shock absorbers on my wheelchair to help me navigate cobblestone roads.

Midori and Jordan found a hotel centrally located near restaurants and shops, in case I wasn't able to travel far in my wheelchair. They booked dining reservations in advance and called ahead to ensure I could get in and out of venues and tables easily. Jordan made inquiries at the Vatican and other museums she hoped we could visit, identifying all the wheelchair-accessible entrances and services ahead of time.

I worried I would be a burden, but everything they had done for me demonstrated how much they all wanted me to go on this trip. They had gone out of their way to make it accessible and comfortable for me. I was overwhelmed with all they had done to make this trip possible.

When I first realized I would be an amputee, one of the things I was most sad about missing was visiting Jordan as she studied abroad. That was something I would never be able to do again, and it caused me such grief to think I wouldn't be there for her on a trip we'd been talking about since her first year of college.

Learning I was going to get to be with Jordan in Rome made me feel like a mom again. It reaffirmed that I was regaining my autonomy and that my kids wanted me to be active in their lives.

Their faith in me was contagious. I could feel myself beginning to step back into my old identity as a capable mother and friend, rather than a helpless victim in constant need of assistance and protection.

One Giant Step

Getting packed for a week away as an amputee was extremely stressful. I obsessively worried I would forget something essential.

How will I navigate a foreign landscape where I don't speak the language and have no idea what kind of accommodations they have for people with mobility issues?

To ease my stress, Scott helped me make a thorough list of the items I might need for the trip. Todd and I packed my suitcase a week in advance, giving us time to discover items we might have missed. I had never been so prepared for a trip.

When the big day arrived, Scott loaded my wheelchair and large suitcase into the back of our car, and I carried the beautiful backpack Midori had given me. It was such a thoughtful gift, providing a place for my passport, lip balm, eyedrops, gum, and a sleep mask, as well as items unique to my new life as an amputee. I had tools to adjust my feet, liner socks to adjust the fit of my prosthetic legs, retractable hiking sticks, and a salve to prevent blisters around my knees and residual limbs. I could hold the backpack in my lap in my wheelchair, then put it over my shoulders to keep my hands free while walking.

I was scared to leave Scott and Todd, but I knew Midori had been with me every step of this journey and would take great care of me in their absence. She had been training for this trip for months. Her enthusiasm and confidence put me at ease.

When we checked in at the ticket counter, the airline attendant summoned someone to escort us in my wheelchair. The escort guided me effortlessly through customs in my wheelchair, helping us through security.

When we got to the security scanners, they asked if I could stand. *Yes I can!* Proudly, I walked through the scanner while my attendant took the wheelchair around to the other side. I was relieved to discover a chair on the other side of the scanner, available for people like me who needed to sit. They performed a security scan on my hands and feet, and once I was cleared, I was assisted back into my wheelchair so I could continue to our flight.

When we got to the gate, we tipped our wheelchair escort, and he left me in Midori's care. Midori assured us both that she would make sure I got onto the plane comfortably. She then checked in with the gate attendant and asked about the procedure to ensure a smooth transfer onto the aircraft so we wouldn't have to worry.

I listened for the announcement about early boarding and realized, for the first time, that in addition to children, they also invite people with disabilities and those who need extra time to board the plane first.

Midori was allowed to accompany me as we boarded the plane with the other passengers who needed extra time. When we got to the plane, I got out of my wheelchair and waited for Midori to help me to my seat. She deftly folded my wheelchair into a travel bag so it could be placed with the other baggage and retrieved upon our arrival in Rome. I put on my backpack so I could hold on to her arm for balance.

A flight attendant explained that a narrow wheelchair was available to help me down the aisle if needed. It was a relief to know that mobility issues like mine weren't unusual for them, and that they were willing and able to help. Still, I wanted to at least try to do it on my own.

We were booked in the first seats closest to the door, so I only had to walk a few steps. After I sat down, we spoke with the flight attendant who had walked with us to our seats to explain my situation. He was excited for me to be traveling and assured me that he would be happy to help me in any way he could.

This was a ten-hour night flight, so I knew I had to get as comfortable as I could. As more passengers boarded the plane, I grew anxious and self-conscious about my legs. I worried about people seeing them, and I didn't know if I should wear my prosthetic sockets or take them off for the flight. And if I did take them off, should I leave the underlying silicone sleeves on my legs, or remove them as I usually did for sleeping? Leaving them on would be uncomfortable, but I was terrified I wouldn't be able to fit back into them in the morning if my legs swelled up while I slept. I had been avoiding salty foods to reduce the risk of swelling, but still, if I couldn't get the silicone sleeves back over my legs, I wouldn't be able to wear my prosthetics to get to the bathroom or exit the plane.

Midori could see that I was anxious and asked me how I was feeling. When I answered honestly, she reminded me that even if I couldn't wear my legs, the flight crew could help get me to a bathroom or to my wheelchair. She assured me she wouldn't leave my side.

"We're going to Rome," she reminded me with a reassuring smile. "We've got this!"

Her excitement was contagious, bringing me back to the present.

I'm sitting on an airplane headed for Europe. Midori and I are going to Italy to see Jordan!

I mentally added "girls' trips" and "international travel" to the growing list of things I could do in my new life after all.

On my first bathroom break, Midori took my arm and walked me there, and waited to help me back to my seat. The next time, I managed it alone, using the walls and the back of the seats to balance.

When I was ready to sleep, I took off my legs and placed them between my seat and Midori's, so nobody would see them. I kept the silicone sleeves on my legs, despite the discomfort. I fretted over what people would think, but nobody seemed to notice. I managed a few hours' sleep before landing in London, where we had to rush to catch a connecting flight.

We had arranged with the airline for me to be escorted in my wheelchair to our connecting gate. We joked that one of the few bonuses of being an amputee was getting to cut security lines and breeze through customs. It was the only part of our trip that was improved because of my amputations. We made it to our connecting gate with time to spare.

I thanked and tipped our companion, and Midori helped me get on the next plane. We were happy with how comfortable our travels had been and confident we could navigate the challenges of wheelchair travel throughout the remainder of the trip. I began to realize that if I would just let myself relax, our week ahead could be an actual vacation rather than a series of obstacles to overcome.

Ciao, Roma!

We checked into our quaint hotel. As requested, they had reserved a room adjacent to the elevator. The bellman said he would bring our bags up and showed us to the elevator that would take us to our first-floor hotel room. The first floor in Europe is one flight above the ground floor.

When the elevator doors opened in the lobby, Midori and I both started laughing as we realized it was the smallest elevator we had ever seen. There was no way we could both fit inside. It was barely large enough to hold my wheelchair.

She maneuvered me inside the elevator, pushed the button for level one, and ran up the stairs to meet me when I arrived. The elevator was as slow as it was small, so when the door opened 30 seconds later, I was greeted with a smiling, if slightly winded, Midori. As promised, our room was just a few steps away.

Anyone who's been to Europe knows that hotel rooms there are relatively small compared to what we're used to in the United States. There was barely room for us to squeeze my wheelchair inside, let alone navigate the room. I would have to stand to get onto the bed and into the bathroom. That was unexpected, but we were pleased to see that they had placed the waterproof chair I had requested in the shower so I could sit while bathing. Rather than getting frustrated, I viewed it as an appropriate challenge for me at this point in my recovery, and incorporated this unintentional obstacle course into my daily physical therapy.

We went out that afternoon to look at nearby shops and had a simple lunch while we waited for Jordan. We'd arranged to meet her a few blocks from our hotel by the river when she finished class. Midori and I enjoyed a stroll through the cobblestone streets, which were easily navigated with the special wheels Scott had installed. As it turns out, there are plenty of people with impaired mobility who live and travel in Italy, so it was more comfortable and accessible than I expected.

The weather was still a bit cool, but the days were sunny, and it felt like spring. Beautiful deciduous trees lined the Tiber River, providing shelter for the many street vendors who set up shops to peddle their art and trinkets to the hordes of tourists visiting Rome and Vatican City.

I couldn't believe I was actually in Italy, about to see my daughter for the first time in three months, and my amputations hadn't stopped this trip from happening.

Finding Persephone

I couldn't wait to see Jordan. Dani had been able to visit us in Seattle over the winter, but Jordan was too far away. I was excited to show her my new walking skills and independence, and to experience Rome through her eyes.

I felt like the goddess Demeter must have felt at the dawning of spring, knowing she would soon be reunited with her beloved Persephone, who had been taken away from her into the underworld for those long, lonely months of winter. I loved the serendipity of our trip being planned for early April, just as winter was fading and spring was blooming. I had spent my winter months recovering, as Dani returned to her new career and Jordan explored the world. Now I was reuniting with Jordan, able to travel and walk for short distances on my new legs.

Just as I had prayed at that altar in Greece 18 months earlier, I had found comfort in the ebb and flow of my girls leading their own lives and coming into my life as they were able. I never could have imagined that our world would be turned upside down and that they would end up caring for me just as I was learning to loosen my reins on them. But life isn't linear.

When we finally saw Jordan walking toward us along the river, we waved and called out excitedly. She ran to us with a massive smile, obviously overjoyed that we had come all this way to be with her.

"You look so healthy!" she exclaimed.

You are so grown up! I thought as we gave each other a huge hug and kiss. There we were: two grown women, both more mature and capable than we'd been the last time we'd seen one another.

I stood up from my wheelchair and took a few steps to show off my new skills. Seeing her amazement at my progress made me realize how far I'd come in just a few months. Seeing myself through her eyes gave me faith in my future. I hoped she could see herself with the love in my eyes as well.

Mangia! Mangia!

That week with Jordan was a whirlwind of exciting experiences. She had made dinner reservations for us every night and had called ahead to the restaurants to ensure we wouldn't be surprised by stairs or obstacles that would be difficult for me to navigate. She attended classes most days, while Midori and I shopped and explored local sights within a mile of our hotel.

Of course, every morning began with my favorite breakfast: a latte and pastry at our cute hotel or a local outdoor *caffè*. Lunches were at small, family-owned osterias and pizzerias in our neighborhood, or closer to Jordan's school, on the chance that she could slip away to meet us. We enjoyed traditional pastas, pizzas, soups, and salads for lunch, saving room for heartier dinners at the restaurants Jordan had chosen.

One restaurant featured delicious truffle, or *tartufo*, in every dish. Another served homemade soups and salads. One waitress went out of her way to give me a soup spoon with a thick, round handle that fit comfortably in my hand with its shortened fingers. She just casually came to the table, replaced my flat spoon, and walked away without saying a word. We were initially confused, then realized she must have seen my hands and wanted to make it easier for me to eat.

This was the first time, other than opening doors or stepping aside, that I had experienced a stranger going out of their way to anticipate how they could make an experience easier for me in my new body. Tears welled up in all of our eyes when Jordan pointed out why she had changed only my spoon. We were all so touched by this thoughtful gesture.

Per our request, Jordan found us a Michelin-starred restaurant as a special celebration for being in Rome together. It had a phenomenal view of the Colosseum. She thought it would be the perfect choice for me since I was too intimidated to tour the famous ruins in my wheelchair.

When she made the reservation, the hostess told Jordan there was a narrow staircase leading up to the main restaurant. Although it was difficult for me to walk up hills with my prosthetic legs, I was able to navigate one or two flights of stairs at a time because each step was flat, so I was standing on solid footing with every step. Knowing that Midori and Jordan would both be there to help me made it easy for me to commit to walking for this special night.

I was anxious about the stairs, but they were relatively easy to ascend, and our table was nearby, per Jordan's request. The view was spectacular as we watched the sun set and the lights come on, illuminating the Colosseum and making the iconic openings glow. It was even more stunning as darkness fell.

As the Michelin stars attest, the food was delicious, beautifully presented, and unique. We were stuffed when they brought course after course of tiny desserts to finish the meal. It was a night we'll remember forever.

Next Steps

That narrow staircase leading up to the restaurant was just a warm-up. In preparation for this trip, I had told Midori my ultimate goal would be to walk up the Spanish Steps before I left Rome. The famous staircase, which leads from the Piazza di Spagna to the church of Trinità del Monti, was near our hotel. We had seen it many times and had taken photos there on multiple occasions while exploring our neighborhood.

The staircase had 135 steps, the equivalent of 11 flights of stairs, which was far more than I had climbed at that point. The stairs were divided into three sections, with small landings between each, symbolizing the holy trinity. It seemed fitting that I would have a chance to rest with The Father, The Son, and The Holy Spirit on my journey up these stairs.

It wasn't lost on me that the three mountains surrounding my

Hanalei home, where I first got sick, were also a trinity in which I had always found comfort.

On our final morning in Rome, in preparation for my big climb, Midori and I ate at a small outdoor caffè near the Piazza di Spagna. This would be my last chance to walk up the Spanish Steps, and I was anxious with anticipation. I had gotten out of my wheelchair to walk to tables in restaurants and to walk around the many small boutiques we had visited, but each of those journeys was only a couple of dozen steps at a time. I worried I wouldn't be able to make it up the Spanish Steps, let alone back down. Midori assured me that I could rest as often as I wanted and could sit down on the steps if I needed to. She reminded me we could always catch a taxi at the top and have it bring us back down as a last resort.

I agreed to give it a try, knowing she would be with me every step of the way if I needed help. I stood up from my wheelchair, and Midori took several photos of me standing at the base of the steps. As I grabbed onto the railing to take my first step, I reminded myself to approach this walk as I had approached my entire recovery: *One tiny step at a time.*

These steps were each a bit higher than my steps at home. I took the first step with my right leg, my dominant one, then brought my left leg up to meet it on that same step. I took the next step with my left leg and was relieved to realize I could lift my body with little difficulty and bring my right leg up to meet my left on the second step. After taking a few steps this way, I began alternating my legs, one leg per step, until I reached the first landing.

I stopped on the first landing and turned around to take in the beautiful view and to look back at all those steps I had just climbed on my own. After a quick rest, I was ready to continue and climb the second set of steps. I ascended that staircase in about half the time it had taken me to climb the first. I celebrated on the second landing with another rest and a chance to see the expanding view that extended farther out into the city as I climbed higher. I charged forward on that third staircase with even more confidence.

I felt such profound faith in my future as I came out on the upper landing of the Spanish Steps and looked back at how far I had come. I had already proven so much to myself on this trip, but ascending these steps on my own was a glimpse into my future and a promise of what it could hold for me.

Midori and I were both elated. Midori had witnessed this journey firsthand from the very beginning. She was there for Dani's frantic phone call and to hear the doctor say that my circulation had been interrupted. She watched my fingers and feet turn purple as hope of saving them waned. She was there with my family when they were told I might not survive, and she prayed with them for my life and my limbs to be saved. She was with me through my surgeries and throughout my recovery. She had been on this entire journey with me, and now she got to see me walking on my own two legs in a city I thought I might never visit. We took dozens of selfies of the two of us standing on that landing with huge smiles on our faces, celebrating what I had done and what I might be able to do in the future.

The future stretched out before me like all those steps I had just climbed – the Piazza di Spagna with its charming fountain below, and all of Rome beyond.

If this is possible, what else is possible? What else can I do that I'd given up hope of ever even attempting?

I would soon discover the real question: *What can I accomplish now that I would never have dared to dream of accomplishing before?ß*

CHAPTER 21

ALOHA AGAIN

"There is nothing like returning to a place that remains unchanged to find the ways in which you yourself have been altered."

– Nelson Mandela

Aloha, Kauai!

Although I felt so fortunate to be recovering in Seattle with extraordinary medical care and my beloved family nearby, I never stopped missing Kauai. After eight months of dedicated recovery, I was ready to face the place of some of my highest highs and lowest lows, with a bit of help from my family and friends.

This time, as I crossed the iconic one-lane bridge into Hanalei, the site of my tearful Jason Mraz moment when I'd first moved there, I wasn't alone: Scott and Todd were with me. I was riding up front, taking in the stunning view that had first made me fall in love with Hanalei. I did my best to hold it together. I could tell Scott and Todd were just as emotional about our return as I was.

"Hey, look at that!" I heard Scott say, pointing to one of the telephone poles poking up out of the tall grass along the river that followed the road into town.

I saw a sign nailed to the pole with a single word painted on it: **"Katy."** As we drove a little farther, I saw the following sign:

"Welcome Home."

The tears that had been welling up began to stream down my cheeks. I'd seen signs like this before, for kids graduating from high school, or on one occasion, welcoming a young man home after an extended hospital stay. But I never thought I'd see *my* name on that telephone pole. I couldn't have asked for a more heartfelt welcome back.

Returning to the Scene of the Crime

As we passed through Hanalei town, I was flooded with memories of raising my kids there in their middle school years and returning for vacations every chance we got through high school and college. When we got to the grocery store, though, I was instantly transported back to the day I arrived from California with that ominous bump on my thumb. I remembered grabbing a thermometer at that same store, wrongly believing it would alert me to a danger I didn't even know was threatening me.

As we turned into our long driveway, my memories bounced between the years of soccer games and visits to the farmer's market, to my last drive home. I looked to Scott and Todd for strength as my mind came back to the present.

When we arrived at the house, Scott and I gave Todd the full tour, showing him the house's layout and the stunning view of the mountains that surround it. When we had gotten ourselves settled, I took them both into our bedroom and told them what I remembered of my lost weekend nine months earlier, when Tiffany saved my life.

The room had changed significantly since I had last been there. We had been planning a remodel when I got sick, so we used our time away as an opportunity to make some changes that would help reframe that room for both of us. We lowered the bathroom floor to remove the three steps where I'd fallen, and moved the bed to a different wall with a big open view of the mountains through a new set of expansive glass doors. The room was barely recognizable, which was a big relief, since I had such traumatic memories of the last time I was there.

Scott, Todd, and I made a pact that, on this trip, we would rewrite the memories of my sepsis experience and reclaim our Hawaiian paradise. But it wasn't easy at first.

Living in My New Skin

I was nervous, being seen in town. I assumed the community had heard what happened, but I also knew that eight months had passed and life had moved on while I was away. Would people even remember me? Would they recognize me in my new form as an amputee? How would they react?

And of course, there are always tourists in a beautiful place like Hanalei, so I knew I would be running into strangers as well as old friends and community members I hadn't seen since my bout with sepsis. How would they feel about being confronted with someone who'd just lost their legs and most of their fingers in idyllic Hawaii?

Do you ever have bad dreams where you're giving a presentation at work or in school, and you suddenly realize you forgot to get dressed, and you're standing there in your underwear? That's how I felt going out in public with my missing limbs on display. It was easier to hide in Seattle and Rome, wearing jeans and long pants. In shorts, I felt like everyone was staring at my prosthetic legs. I felt so uncomfortable that when I would pay for something, I would hide my fingers under my credit card, with my normal-looking thumb on top, so as not to call attention to my missing fingertips and unsettle those around me.

Over and over again, I caught myself masking and minimizing my presence, making myself small in ways I never had before. I was trying to blend in, to hide in plain sight.

Over time, though, as more and more people recognized me and welcomed me back with genuine joy and warmth, I began to feel normal again. More like my prior self and less like an oddity. As friends gathered to meet Todd and thank him for taking such good care of me, and to toast my survival and recovery, I found it increasingly difficult to keep playing small and dulling my shine. Maybe I didn't remember who I was, or how fearless I had once been, but they did. My body had changed, but my friends reminded me that I was still me.

Back to My Beach

Bolstered by the way the community treated me – not as a frail amputee, but as the Katy they had always known and loved – I decided I was ready to tackle the goal I'd been dreaming of for eight long months: going back to my favorite beach for a swim.

When I lived on Kauai, this beautiful beach would often call to me to play on its shore and in its waves. I loved going there and had so many special memories of swimming with my kids when they were young, and collecting sunrise shells after storms. It was the beach I'd pictured as my fondest memory of Hawaii when the air ambulance flew me to Seattle. That day, I promised myself I would return there when I recovered.

For eight months, I had dedicated myself to that recovery, envisioning a future in which my body could handle what I had come to think of as my amputee triathlon: the treacherous hike down to the beach, the walk through the deep sand, and the wade into the waves for the ultimate reward of a real ocean swim.

Back when I had a hard time believing I would actually walk again, it was an act of faith to imagine I might one day be able to navigate that rugged path and swim in the chaotic currents of the Pacific Ocean. But now that I had been to Rome and back, I felt like anything was possible.

Look for the Helpers

I was able to drive my truck with my prosthetic legs up to the trailhead at the top of the hill that led down to the beach. Our friend Emily met Scott and me there with an ATV that Scott borrowed to drive me down the steep trail to the sand below. I felt such joy and freedom stepping off the ATV onto the beach with my new legs, holding Scott's arm as we walked through the deep sand toward the water.

There were about 20 people on the beach that day. Their stares made me feel self-conscious about my metal legs, my pale skin, and my scarred, bikini-clad body.

Although I knew I looked like a visitor to the island with my pale skin and short hair, my familiar beach was welcoming me home. As the other beachgoers got used to my presence, I started to relax and feel like one of them, just another person enjoying a lovely day of white sand and steady surf.

I knew I wanted to swim, but in my own time. I encouraged Scott to get some exercise by swimming laps just offshore and told Emily to go ahead and follow her son into the nearby tidepool, assuring them that I would be fine. With my loved ones distracted, I awkwardly walked the few steps to the water where I could privately relax in the shallow waves.

Finally being back in these magical waters was the most delicious feeling imaginable. The warm, blue-gray waves washing onto my new body felt accepting and loving. They beckoned me deeper into the water.

A young couple who had been sitting next to me on the sand were swimming nearby, so I felt safe to scoot out a little deeper to walk in the waves. I was comfortable walking as the buoyant salt water supported my body, so I decided to lift my legs and float on the shallow waves. Knowing I wasn't totally alone, with the young couple playing right next to me, I went ahead and let myself go a little deeper to feel the freedom of floating. I practiced kicking my legs and moving my arms in the salty seawater. It was sublime.

Just as I was feeling my most confident, swimming in about six feet of water, one of my prosthetic legs slipped off. I looked down and watched in horror as it floated to the ocean floor beneath me. Reflexively, I plugged my nose to try to dive after it, but realized that my body was so buoyant, and my half-leg and prosthetic leg were so ineffective at kicking, I was unable to leave the surface. It felt like I was wearing a life vest.

I tried a second time, to no avail. I felt a little like the Disney/Pixar character, Nemo, swimming in circles with his one good fin and his partial "lucky" fin.

In desperation, I called out to the young man nearby, trying to find the right words to describe my situation without startling him or scaring him off.

"Excuse me," I said, "I'm so sorry to bother you, but I…um... I was swimming here just now when one of my prosthetic legs fell off and sank to the bottom. It's right beneath me, just a few feet down, but I can't reach it. Would you mind diving for it and returning it to me?"

I looked between him and his girlfriend, who by that time was standing in the water near the shore, and stared into some of the biggest, most shocked and concerned eyes I had ever seen.

The young man assured me he'd be happy to help, as his girlfriend looked on anxiously. The look in her eyes told me she was counting on him to handle this delicate situation with the utmost chivalry.

As he began swimming my way to get my leg for me, my second prosthetic leg fell off and sank to the bottom, and I was left with my stubby legs kicking ineffectually beneath me, 10 feet from the shore. If I felt helpless with one leg missing, I now felt completely ridiculous at having lost *both* of my legs.

Out of habit, I was kicking to try to get closer to shore, but the only result was exhaustion. No forward progress whatsoever. I could feel the mounting pressure this young man was under to be my personal savior in my time of need.

I looked around to realize it was not just his girlfriend who was counting on him to save my prosthetic legs, but everyone else on the beach who had just watched me walk down to the water by myself. Twenty pairs of eyes watched us with rapt attention as I used my strong arms to swim for the shore while the young woman walked deeper into the ocean to help me out of the water. When I got about halfway to her, my helpful hero emerged out of the water with *both* of my legs.

It all happened so quickly that I reflexively reached out to take my legs from him. It was at that moment, as my head sank below the surface, that it became clear to all of us that I was only able to swim because of my arms; my little legs were helpless beneath me. Just as my head began to go underwater, I shoved the prosthetic legs back into his hands and continued to swim desperately for the shore.

His girlfriend ran out to meet me while he kicked his legs frantically to keep his head above the water as he carried my waterlogged prostheses in both of his hands. I awkwardly scooted up onto the sand, being careful not to meet the eyes of any gawkers on the shore. Although I was able to distract Emily and Scott so that I could enter the water on my own, I had forgotten about the beach full of people who couldn't take their eyes off me.

On that day, a beautiful day at my special beach, I learned firsthand the true meaning of compassion, humility, and community. In that brief moment, my moment of need, when I looked toward that beach from the water, I saw 20 people ready to jump into the ocean to make sure I made it safely to shore.

Sometimes, when I think back on that day, I start to feel bad for the young couple who got drawn into my story. But then I giggle, remembering that I gave them one of the most unique stories of something discovered in the ocean: two prosthetic legs and a mermaid with two lucky fins!

CHAPTER 22

SOLID FOOTING

"And one day she discovered that she was fierce, and strong, and full of fire, and that not even she could hold herself back because her passion burned brighter than her fears."

– Mark Anthony

I was standing in line to get a cup of coffee, prosthetic legs on full display below my skirt, when a woman behind me leaned over to her companion and whispered with palpable excitement, "That's Katy Grainger!"

Hearing a stranger excited to see me in public was not something I'd ever expected to happen. I suppose the same could be said of nearly every experience I'd had since that purple bump first appeared on my thumb five years earlier. But that moment? That was something special.

It happened at a conference for an international diagnostics company held in Mexico. Even before that lovely moment of recognition, the entire experience had already been a dream come true. The company requested *me* to be a keynote speaker. They'd contacted

Sepsis Alliance, which acted as my agent, negotiating a substantial fee that solidified my status as a professional speaker.

I was thrilled to be paid enough to not only cover my expenses but also to make a significant donation to Sepsis Alliance. I felt acknowledged for the years of hard work I had put into becoming a sepsis and disability educator, a storyteller, a patient advocate, and a public speaker. I had given many paid talks before, but at this event, I officially recognized myself as the professional speaker and patient advocate I had become.

At the conference, I was treated like a VIP at every turn: flown to Cancun, met by a driver, booked into a stunning hotel room, then ushered to the green room. There, a professional stylist did my hair and makeup, and a tech crew placed a wireless mic on my lapel before escorting me to the stage.

If stepping out onto that stage with a packed house of 2,000 people cheering me on wasn't enough to convince me that my story was resonating, that woman leaning over to her friend a few hours later and whispering my name sure was.

How did I get here?

The Road to Recognition

Unlike sepsis, it didn't happen overnight.

Let's rewind to 2019. By August of that year, 11 months after falling ill, I'd finally reached a point in my recovery where I no longer needed regular in-home care. Honestly, Scott and I could have gotten along on our own sooner, but Todd was so helpful that we had a hard time letting him go. Over the prior months, he slowly tapered his hours, helping me realize I was ready to face life on my own. We said a grateful farewell to the wonderful man who had become like a member of our family, and faced the challenge of everyday life without his help.

I thought it was a coincidence at the time, but I now realize that Dani had carefully orchestrated leaving her job that September to spend the fall and winter holidays in the Seattle area one last time before she permanently moved to Hawaii to start a family with Hunter.

I will be forever grateful for the 15 months of loving support I received from Todd and my family!

Not All Superheroes Wear Capes

In September of 2019, as the first anniversary of my sepsis nightmare approached, I participated in a Sepsis Alliance fundraiser called the Sepsis Superhero Challenge. Their website encourages participants to "go the extra mile to raise sepsis awareness and honor those affected by sepsis."

The Sepsis Superhero Challenge was an ideal opportunity to support Sepsis Alliance and thank them for saving lives through education, and supporting families who've experienced sepsis. It was also a great chance to show my friends and family how well I was recovering, and challenge myself to literally "go the extra mile" by walking my first full mile as an amputee. It was empowering to see how far I'd come in a year and to be able to help others once again.

I could feel the tide turning, but I never could have imagined where that one-mile walk would take me. Not only did I complete the walk-a-thon, but my donations caught the attention of Sepsis Alliance. When they reached out to thank me, I was invited to meet their CEO, Thomas Heymann, who would be visiting Seattle a few weeks later for a sepsis conference.

Dani and I met him at a coffee shop, where he asked me about my experience with sepsis. I shared all I had been through and thanked him for the information and support we found on the Sepsis Alliance website throughout my journey. He appreciated my enthusiasm, and he shared more about the programs and services Sepsis Alliance could provide, thanks to grassroots fundraisers and donations like mine. As he shook my hand when we parted ways, he said he'd like to keep in touch.

An Answer to a Long-Ago Prayer

A week later, Thomas reached out and invited me to apply for a position on the Sepsis Alliance Board of Directors. I was flattered, and thrilled to have the opportunity to help an organization working to reduce suffering and harm caused by sepsis.

I never could have predicted the circuitous route it would take, but the purpose I'd been seeking since my kids left home, and praying about for years, had finally arrived. I officially became a Sepsis Alliance board member in January of 2020.

COVID-19

Three months later, a trip to California with an invitation to share my patient experience was cancelled due to a mysterious viral infection that was spreading like wildfire. I flew to Hawaii instead, where we hosted Jordan and her 10 college housemates for spring break of their senior year. The COVID-19 pandemic was declared just days after the girls returned to their families at the end of the week. Classes were moved online, the state of Hawaii suspended flights, we watched Jordan's college graduation ceremony online with our immediate family, and the Class of 2020 received their diplomas by mail.

I made a few short videos for Sepsis Alliance that were posted on their social media and attended monthly online Board meetings. I learned as much as I could about sepsis. The more I learned, the more I noticed the similarities between what I had experienced and what patients with COVID-19 were dealing with.

I had continual anxiety, and experienced PTSD when I heard about lungs failing, patients being intubated, overcrowded ICUs, lack of available life-saving equipment, and death numbers increasing daily. I cried for the patients who were isolated from their families. If my family had not been with me to give me the will to fight and to help me breathe in my early days, I know I would have died. I felt survivor's guilt for having quality care and availability of resources that kept me alive just 18 months earlier. This was a traumatic time, but it fueled my passion to help save lives.

As I suspected, more and more evidence began to support my gut instinct that many of the patients whose deaths were attributed to COVID-19 were actually due to viral sepsis (sepsis caused by the viral infection COVID-19). In June of 2020, as a member of the National Institute of Health's (NIH) COVID-19 Guidelines Panel, Steve Simpson, the Medical Director of Sepsis Alliance, and Angel Coz, a Sepsis Alliance Advisory Board member, were among the first to publish findings that deaths from COVID-19 were indeed caused by sepsis. Sepsis explained why, although many people recovered, a small percentage became extremely sick with a seemingly dysregulated response to infection and organ failure: hallmarks of sepsis. Over the next few years, an increasing number of peer-reviewed studies supported these findings.

Using my Voice for the Limb-Loss and Limb-Difference Community

During the COVID-19 pandemic, I also began making connections in the amputee community. I attended virtual meetings with the Amputee Coalition[1] and Enhancing Skills For Life (ESFL,)[2] an organization that supports people living without both hands or all four limbs. Both organizations support the limb-loss and limb-difference community. Although I'm not missing my hands, my missing fingers qualify as partial hand loss, so I consider myself a "quad amputee," a person missing parts of all four limbs. Both groups have welcomed me with open hearts.

---

1. Amputee Coalition empowers people with limb loss and limb difference through resources, support, and advocacy.
2. SFL's mission is to educate, empower, and connect those living without both hands, both arms, or all four limbs.

Amputee Coalition's resources educated my family and me about becoming an amputee, and their annual conference allowed me to attend workshops, see products designed for the limb-loss community, and make friends from all over the country. At their events, I attended training sessions where I learned to run, swim, bike, play pickle ball, and use adaptive devices to prepare food. They even taught me how to fall safely so I wouldn't break a bone if I lost my balance. I did advanced training to become a Certified Peer Visitor to support new amputees and became a Lead Advocate in my state, including going to Washington DC to advocate for the limb-loss and limb-difference communities. I'm still in regular contact with the friends I made, and we meet annually at the Amputee Coalition National Conference.

Through my friends in the amputee community, I was introduced to Enhancing Skills For Life, which opened my eyes to the unique and important needs of the upper-limb-loss community. I have learned more tips and tricks about doing things differently with the loss of my fingers than I could have imagined. With the guidance of my peers in this group, and an invaluable list of adaptive devices, I have learned to function effortlessly with the loss of my fingers. Both groups helped me through my difficult first few years as an amputee, and now I volunteer with them as often as I can.

An Anniversary to Remember

Nine months later, after telling shortened versions of my sepsis story in several articles, podcasts, and news profiles, I was asked to give the keynote speech at the Sepsis Alliance Summit, two years to the day after I was admitted to the hospital in septic shock.

Knowing that speech would be delivered on the second anniversary of my most significant trauma was much more emotionally challenging than I'd anticipated. As the Summit approached, each passing day brought a fresh batch of reminders of what my friends, family, and I had been through two years before.

I faced the challenge of writing and delivering a detailed, high-profile speech the same way I faced my recovery: one tiny step at a time.

Combing methodically through my experience, I described my symptoms, the medical interventions that saved my life, and the warning signs to look for, in hopes that nobody who heard me speak would have to go through what I had experienced.

My speech was pre-recorded, so I was able to film it in advance without the added stress of delivering it live on my sepsis anniversary. A week later, on the date my life changed forever, Scott and I watched my talk online with 1,500 other participants. We sat hand in hand on the couch where I had recovered from my amputations, streaming the conference on our TV.

As I watched myself speak, I saw my story through the eyes of someone who had never heard it before. At the same time, I relived it. It was extremely emotional for me to see the pain on my face and hear the cracking in my voice as I recalled the events that nearly cost me my life and ended up making me a multiple amputee. I cried for myself. I cried for Scott and my family. I cried for others impacted by sepsis. I was so grateful that, after all I had gone through, my story was being used to educate others about sepsis and improve sepsis recognition, treatment, and care.

I was no longer overwhelmed by sepsis; I had taken back the narrative of my life and was using my experience to enact change. For the past two years, my life had felt unstable. But the love and support of my family, and my work with Sepsis Alliance, had given me back the solid footing I had been fighting to regain.

Standing Up to Sepsis

A week later, as I felt myself surfing over the waves of my grief rather than drowning in them, it seemed appropriate to stand-up paddle for a mile as my second annual Sepsis Superhero Challenge fundraiser. The prior year, I'd used my new legs to walk a mile; this year, I would use my hands to grip the paddle that propelled me forward while balancing on an oversized surfboard. My friends and family have continued to help raise awareness by participating with me and making generous donations to Sepsis Alliance.

Every year, I've tried to keep raising the bar on my Sepsis Superhero Challenge Fundraiser by changing my activity to showcase the improvements in my abilities as a multiple amputee. In year three, after re-learning how to snowboard that winter, I went wakesurfing for a mile to show off the strength of my hands and my improved balance. In year four, I traveled back to Greece and walked a mile up the rustic cliffside steps to the church featured in the film *Mamma Mia!*, to demonstrate my confidence in traveling and my ability to hike and climb with the help of friends. In the past few years, I've walked a mile in Washington, DC, meeting with senators and representatives, educating about sepsis and amputations, and asking for support on bills that could help the sepsis and amputee communities.

Losing an Angel

As I was finally putting my sepsis trauma behind me and reclaiming a new life, tragedy struck again.

"I have some tough news," Heidi warned me, on what I had thought was just a check-in phone call.

I took a deep breath. "What is it?" I asked, steeling myself for whatever she had to say. My thoughts immediately went to Heidi's family. Her mom had been sick. I really hoped nothing had happened to her.

"Todd died," she said gravely.

"Todd who?" I wondered if that was her uncle, whom I had met years before when we were kids. They had been really close.

"Nurse Todd," she said gently, trying to help me understand.

It took me a minute to realize she meant *my* Todd.

"Oh my God. No! What happened?" I asked, as tears filled my eyes.

"He had a sudden, massive heart attack," Heidi explained, "the kind they call a widowmaker. It happened so suddenly, he probably didn't even realize it was happening."

I was stunned. Todd had sent me a text a week earlier, saying he'd seen my keynote speech online and was cheering me on. And I had just listened to a voice message from him on my birthday, a few days earlier. I hadn't had a chance to call him back. My heart sank, realizing I would never get that chance now.

That voice message will forever be saved on my phone as a reminder of one of my best friends:

"I'm calling to wish you Happy Birthday! I hope you are sleeping in. The only thing better than it being your birthday is if it were my birthday, but it's your turn to be the Queen of Everything, so I will pass my tiara to you. I love you very much! I hope you are hanging out with family, surrounded by love and knowing that you are loved. Happy Birthday. Thank you for being a gift to my life and so many other people's lives by just being born and just being you. Happy Birthday!"

I listen to his message on my birthday every year and can still feel his love, sense of humor, and generosity.

Todd told me many times in the course of our time together that his father had passed away in his early 50's, so he lived each day as though it were his last. I never imagined the same thing would happen to him. I'm sure he didn't either.

He was one of the most fun, carefree people I knew. His sunny personality was contagious, uplifting everyone he met, even those going through the most challenging times of their lives. He had been an angel in my life, a gift from God to help my family and me heal. I know I wasn't alone in feeling that way, because he'd told me about the many friends he still kept in touch with whom he met in his work as their private nurse. He had found his true calling, and the world was a better place because of him.

Heidi went on, "Michael would really like to see you. He knows how special your time with Todd was, and he wants to be with you right now."

I was deeply touched to be invited by Todd's husband to share memories and grieve together in person.

"Yes, of course! I would love that."

The Rainbow Connection

The lunch Michael and I shared a week later was wonderful. It felt like we'd been friends for ages, rather than having greeted each other only briefly. We swapped stories and shared memories of our time with Todd while enjoying a nice lunch at one of Michael's favorite restaurants.

When we left the restaurant, a light rain was falling: a typical winter day in Seattle. As we walked under the shops' eaves, we noticed people pointing up at the sky and taking pictures. We followed their collective gaze and found ourselves staring, open-mouthed, at a magnificent double rainbow stretching across the Seattle sky, looking as if it ended right in front of us in the parking lot of University Village.

We looked at each other, tears streaming down our faces, and said in unison, "It's Todd!"

There was no doubt in either of our minds. Todd had sent two rainbows, one for each of us, to let us know he loved us and would continue to look out for us from beyond.

Influencing Sepsis Awareness

The confirmation of that feeling that Todd still had my back came just a few days later, when I got a call from Tom Heymann, saying the video of my keynote speech from the Sepsis Alliance Summit was blowing up on YouTube. I didn't even know Sepsis Alliance had posted it online.

"It already has 10,000 views," he declared.

That got my attention. Over the next few weeks, I watched in astonishment as that number grew by about a thousand views a day. Hundreds of people left comments, and I did my best to respond to each one as quickly as possible.

"Thank you, Todd!" I whispered as I saw the number of views climb into *six figures* over the next few weeks, "Whatever you're doing to help me spread the word about sepsis, it's working."

That video has remained popular and has now been seen by over half a million people worldwide. That's a lot of views for a 35-minute video about someone getting sick!

People were genuinely fascinated by my story. People who had experienced loss or trauma felt inspired and less alone. People who didn't know about sepsis were learning the symptoms and sharing the information with friends and family. Fellow sepsis survivors and amputees saw me as a peer and even a friend.

By telling my truth, I was saving lives.

Over the years, I've heard from numerous people that my story encouraged them or a loved one to get medical help in early sepsis before it became serious or deadly. In person and online, I've also been given the opportunity to support many people through the recovery process from sepsis and/or amputations. Through my experience, they've been inspired to lead productive new lives.

"Like it or not, you're now officially an influencer, Auntie Katy," my nephew Darrick declared with a smile one morning over coffee.

He was half joking, but I knew he wasn't wrong. *What was I supposed to do with this platform I'd been given?*

I had prayed for a purpose, but I never imagined how big my purpose might become. It was clear from the encouragement the world was giving me that I was being called to do even more. When I doubted myself, I thought of all I had already accomplished that I never could have imagined. I committed to seeking guidance from experts to explore possibilities for my future, excited to see what new opportunities might lie ahead.

Finding Meaning in My Story

While battling sepsis, even when I didn't know what was happening to me, I knew two things: I wanted to reclaim my health and life, and I wanted to spread sepsis awareness so others wouldn't have to become as sick as I was. But from the comments on the YouTube video, I could see that my story was touching different people for different reasons. So many people were relating to me: sepsis survivors, people who lost loved ones to sepsis, amputees, older women, doctors, nurses, pharmaceutical manufacturers, medical device manufacturers, prosthetists, cancer survivors, people with paralysis or rare diseases… the list goes on.

How could I have the most significant impact with my story? What was I meant to be to these groups of people?

I needed help.

Darrick introduced me to Dr. Adrienne MacIain, Memoir Midwife, who helped me become a better speaker, storyteller, and influencer. Together, we clarified who my story was for and the journey it would take them on. We found the emotional arc of the story, rather than getting hung up on chronology and technical details that would sail right over the heads of a non-medical audience.

But most importantly, we discovered the person I wanted to be in the world, empowering me to show up authentically in each new moment.

Later, when I realized I needed help and support in writing my book, I knew right away who to reach out to. Adrienne knew my story, understood my needs, and had not only the right skill set, but the right energy to help bring my book to life.

As my social media following grew, I quickly realized I needed someone to help me manage my public online presence. I posted on my private Facebook page for close friends and family, asking if anyone knew a high school student who wanted to be my Social

Media Manager in exchange for community service hours and a college reference.

I was significantly underestimating my need, but fortunately, I got an immediate response from Jessica "Jes" Tuffield, a sepsis survivor and patient advocate from England with whom I had connected online. She had a large following in the sepsis community, and I looked to her as a role model of what my advocacy could become.

When she reached out to me, I was both flattered and scattered. I told her I didn't really know what I needed. Undeterred, she simply replied, "I'm your gal!" That she was, and still is.

As a fellow sepsis survivor, Jes shared my passion for sepsis awareness and immediately grasped my mission and vision. She had been a sepsis advocate for years and was looking for an opportunity to reach more people. My new popularity was the perfect opportunity for both of us. Between her media savvy and my visibility, our Facebook and Instagram following has grown significantly, and continues to climb.

As more and more speaking opportunities poured in – *Women's Health* Magazine, New York State Office for the Aging, World Sepsis Congress, *Amplitude* Magazine, etc. – I continued to hone my skills and grow my confidence. I started getting invited on podcasts, including *The Bravest Kind*, *PodcastDX*, and the extremely popular *This Podcast Will Kill You*, which averages two million listens per episode.

In September of 2021, I gave the closing speech at the Sepsis Alliance Summit. The following July, I was invited to speak on an amputee panel for a webinar for an exciting new project called Sepsis Alliance Connect, a virtual support community for people affected by sepsis. I had been passionate about this project since I'd joined the Sepsis Alliance Board, and was thrilled to provide information for their extensive online resource library.

It was finally starting to sink in that I was no longer just a survivor: I was a subject-matter expert making a real impact.

Dancing through Life

After I became aware that I was going to lose my fingertips and lower legs, I began to mourn all of the things I thought I would no longer be able to do, like walking, running, and writing my name. But harder still was mourning the things I thought I would never *get* to do, things I'd been looking forward to all my life. Little did I know then that I would still have the chance to do those things, just not quite in the way I'd once imagined.

In May of 2022, I was overjoyed to walk down the aisle and dance at Dani and Hunter's wedding as we gained a fabulous son-in-law. My prosthetic legs had adjustable feet, allowing me to walk in and out of the wedding ceremony in high-heeled gold Gucci sandals that beautifully matched my mother-of-the-bride gown. After the ceremony, I snuck away and slipped on new white leather tennis shoes that were perfectly hidden beneath the hem of my gown. For the rest of the night, I could move more freely and even dance, holding onto the hands of my partners for balance. I was so grateful to be there to celebrate the expansion of our family.

Two years later I would again be mother of the bride at Jordan and Kai's wedding on Whidbey Island outside of Seattle. Again, I danced and celebrated as I always dreamed I would.

I was still dancing through life, even on prosthetic legs.

September 2022 - Skopelos, Greece

On the eve of my 4th sepsis anniversary, I found myself sitting on a gorgeous balcony on the island of Skopelos, looking out over the aquamarine Aegean Sea, contemplating how much my life had changed in just a few short years.

I was once again hosted by Jeannette, the same friend who had invited me five years earlier. She had gone out of her way to ensure accommodations for my new physical needs. We would not move from town to town as we had on the last trip. This time, we would begin in Athens, where Jeannette would arrange an elevator ride to the top of the Acropolis so I could revisit the Parthenon, a place I had fallen in love with on my first trip and feared I might never get to experience again.

We would then travel by bus and boat to the stunning island of Skopelos. We would stay in a beautiful oceanfront hotel for a week and Jeannette would show us all the best places, as she had moved to the island from California a few years earlier. This was an intention she had set on our last journey to Greece.

Receiving her invitation allowed me to dream of new possibilities for my life. I never imagined I'd return to Greece. With Scott's blessing, I accepted the offer to join her and a group of other women seeking time away to contemplate our lives. I reached out to Midori, who had been struggling with a transition of her own: retiring from a job she'd held for over 20 years. She was intrigued by the possibility of experiencing the kind of transformation and renewal I'd had on my first visit to Greece, and Midori took the trip as the excuse she'd been looking for to leave work and move on to the next phase of her life.

She and I embarked on this journey together, just as we had four years prior in the hospital on Kauai, and again a few months later when we visited Jordan in Rome. But this time, the wheelchair that escorted me through the airport was an option I could choose if I needed a little help, rather than a necessity I couldn't avoid. I proudly rode in the airport's wheelchair, escorted across the concourse with full appreciation for the accommodations available for people with difficulty getting around. I was grateful to have learned to navigate these accommodations, and that my sweet angel Midori, who came to my aid when I needed her most, could be there to witness how far I'd come.

The highlight of that trip was hosting my annual Sepsis Superhero Challenge Fundraiser there, reliving a scene from *Mamma Mia!*, one of my favorite movies. I hiked down a steep hill to the ocean, across a narrow land bridge, and up the uneven steps carved into the rock outcropping that houses Agios Ioannis Kastri, the church where the wedding in the movie took place. When I arrived at the top, I was cheered on by my fellow travelers as I rang a celebratory bell in the tiny chapel and lit candles in memory of Todd.

I felt a deeply rooted confidence I hadn't experienced in years. The writing and soul-searching we did in our workshops on the trip inspired me to imagine new possibilities for my life. I realized it was time to commit to writing my book. The island offered me a refuge to begin the dreaming phase of my writing process. It was the ideal place to step outside of my experience and watch it begin to take shape. With hindsight, I could finally see it for the story it had become: I was so much more than just the trauma I had survived. My story represented hope, healing, passion, and purpose.

Model Behavior

After returning from my second Greek odyssey, I was treated to yet another experience I never thought I'd have: my first professional modeling gig, as an amputee in my 50's!

Thanks to a recommendation from the photographer who shot photos for my website, Rad Power Bikes hired me to be featured in an online commercial for their new RadTrike. My contract gave them full usage rights to my images, but I never expected the text I received from my sister-in-law Holly, with a photo showing a *nine-foot* window decal of my image at the entrance to Rad Power Bikes in Salt Lake City.

On a whim, I drove by the Seattle location and found my image plastered on the front of that store too. It was deeply validating to be treated as model material and to have the opportunity to normalize disability in such a public way.

A Mother's Love

My family was excited to see me happy and fulfilled with my varied endeavors. At the same time I did the Rad Power Bikes ad, I was volunteering passionately with Sepsis Alliance, sharing my story on social media, and had procured an interview in a local magazine to discuss sepsis, amputations, and how I had gotten my life back on track. Nobody was prouder of me than my mom.

During my recovery, she told me so many times that she wished she could trade places with me, I lost count. I'll never forget that, early in my recovery, she even wondered if there was a way to give her fingers to me if I were to lose mine. I can't imagine what it must have been like for her to see the sweet baby she had given birth to nearly die, and then lose those perfect little feet and fingertips she had counted on the day I was born. We're never too old to be our parents' babies.

Every time I saw her over the years, I caught a glimpse of sadness in her eyes before she put on a smile when she realized I was thriving and that she was happy we could be together. She never missed an opportunity to tell me how proud she was. In fact, on Facebook, an app she rarely used before I got sick, she was my number one supporter and often the first to comment on my daily posts. But as babies age, so do parents. She had been slowing down in her early 80's when I got sick, but her health was good right up until she got a diagnosis of metastatic cancer and was given "days to weeks" to live.

In December of 2022, less than two weeks after her diagnosis, my mother passed away from, of all things, *sepsis* caused by a cancer-related infection. The force of the emotional blow of losing my mother sent me reeling, reigniting the initial sepsis trauma from which I had never fully healed. Not emotionally, anyway.

I realized that in my rush to heal my body, move on with my life, and start sharing my story with the world, I hadn't allowed myself the time I needed to emotionally heal. As I processed my mother's death, I made the tough decision to set the book aside for a while and refocus on self-care and my own holistic healing. How could I tell my authentic story when I was still grieving the loss of my mother and wasn't fully healed?

At first, I judged myself harshly for considering putting the book project on hold, but I could feel my mom's love, and Todd's too, reminding me to listen to my body and take care of myself. I needed to heed my own advice and take two steps back in my recovery to give myself time to fully heal so I could move forward.

Pausing the writing of my book allowed me time to continue with my volunteer work and sepsis awareness, while allowing me time to journal more, seek therapy for my mental recovery, and focus on my personal life – all things I had been neglecting. I knew my mom would be proud of this decision because, more than anyone, she just wanted me to take care of myself and be happy.

A week after putting all of my book research deep into a file on my desk, I received a copy of the magazine with my recent interview. To my astonishment, the editor chose to put me on the cover of the magazine, showing off my prosthetic legs, looking strong, confident, and empowered. As with the thousands of YouTube views I felt Todd had somehow orchestrated after his passing, I believed my mom had a hand in this. To this day, I still feel her cheering me on in all I do.

"Isn't TikTok Just a Dancing Platform?"

I'd been hearing from Jes for a while that I should give TikTok a try as a way to spread sepsis awareness to a new audience. I was skeptical at first because I only knew it as the dance app for bored teenagers that became popular during the COVID-19 pandemic.

Sure enough, when I first started scrolling through TikTok right before New Year's Eve in 2021, I mostly saw dance videos and things that would appeal to a younger audience. But after I began clicking the "like" button on content from older creators, and seeking out medical and amputee content, the algorithm started sending me videos that were more appealing to me and more like the ones I wanted to create.

TikTok is like YouTube, but with short videos in a mobile-only format. They had just started allowing three-minute videos, up from one minute, so it was a space where I could easily share short stories about sepsis awareness and life as an amputee.

I went ahead and ripped off the Band-Aid by posting a 15-second video of a baby shark swimming in front of our house in Hawaii, adding a couple of stickers, and playing the popular "Baby Shark" song in the background. Right away, it started getting likes and comments. I was amazed at how easy it was to engage with people on the app.

I decided to try another one. This time, I took a 15-second video of my prosthetic legs and feet, relaxing in my classic Hawaiian hammock with the ocean beyond. I layered in some tropical music and posted it.

Just as I'd hoped, the contrast of my prosthetic legs against that idyllic background intrigued people. It got a few hundred views, and I gained a few followers. They wanted to know what had happened, but even more than that, they wanted to know who this woman was, living her best life despite such a devastating loss.

I started making longer videos in more of a storytelling format. I wanted to grow my following and video views so the TikTok algorithm would keep pushing my videos to new people so I could reach more people with sepsis education. Then I got more strategic, planning to release a series telling my whole sepsis and amputation story in three-minute chunks, each ending with a cliffhanger.

Six weeks later, during Sepsis Survivor Week in mid-February, I began making videos from Hanalei, where I first got sepsis. I filmed the first one at the airport, where I discovered the bump on my finger. I made the second one in the parking lot of the walk-in clinic I first went to, and the third one was at my house in Hanalei. I wanted to simulate the experience from the locations where it all happened. It was healing for me and seemed like a compelling way to tell the story. I recorded and edited four videos that day.

It worked! I posted the first videos that night before I went to bed, and woke up to my videos blowing up, with several thousand views and people begging for the rest of the story. I was gaining thousands of views every hour as I scrambled to film the remaining parts of the story.

By the time I'd finished the entire story, my following had ballooned to over 35,000 people! I was shocked to realize there was a place on TikTok for a disabled woman in her 50's, and heartened to know that so many strangers cared about my story, and sepsis and disability awareness.

Thank You for Saving My Life

In January of 2023, I had the opportunity to return to The Queen's Medical Center to thank the medical team that saved my life. It was an incredible experience to meet the people who had so profoundly impacted my life. Although I barely remembered most of them because I had been so sick when they treated me, they all remembered me and were visibly touched to see how well I was doing. It was a rare opportunity for them to see the fruits of all their hard work.

Just like in that dream I'd had in that same hospital five years earlier, there I was, surrounded by my medical team as they applauded, cheered, and offered me congratulatory hugs. I had done it! Or rather, we had, as a team. Against all odds, we had won, and now we were finally getting the chance to celebrate that hard-earned victory.

To my surprise, there was a news crew there to document the reunion, which was broadcast statewide on Hawaii News Now. They filmed my triumphant return, as well as interviews with me and several of my doctors from The Queen's Medical Center on Oahu. Through my story, the residents of Hawaii were learning about the dangers of untreated infections and the symptoms of sepsis.

A few months later, I was invited back to give a keynote speech at a dinner hosted by The Queen's Health Systems. I stood on a stage, holding the rapt attention of the 400 medical professionals in the room, sharing my story as an example of all the patients whose lives they had saved. It was a deeply powerful experience for all involved.

A Call for Help

While I was in Honolulu for that talk, I got a phone call from my neighbor in Hanalei. The 52-year-old wife of a friend of his was in the ICU at Queen's with septic shock, fighting for her life. It gave me chills that her situation was almost identical to mine.

"If she lives, she may lose limbs," he told me.

My heart broke for this couple, going through what we'd been through. Though I wasn't able to visit her right away since she was still in the ICU, I was able to meet her husband at the hospital and give him encouragement and advice.

I watched him descend the hospital staircase, disheveled and exhausted, and had the uncanny feeling I was watching my own husband through a time portal. When he spoke, it was Scott's voice I heard, saying, "I don't know what to do. My wife's going to wake up, and her hands and feet are so damaged, and I'm just… I just want her to live. That's all I want. I want her to *live*, and I want her to *want* to live."

I saw this man take in my prosthetic legs and missing fingers, first with the usual discomfort, but eventually with hope as he commented on how vibrantly alive and well-adapted to my new body I was.

"We found you online, and we've been trying to learn from your story," he told me, as we stood in the hall outside the ICU. "It's been really helpful, but this is all just so…" He gestured in a way that clearly conveyed total overwhelm.

"I know," I reassured him, "and it's going to feel that way for a while. Just when you think you're through the hard part, you realize the real challenges are just getting started. But there is life after sepsis, and it's worth living."

A couple of weeks later, I made another trip to Oahu to visit Diane and her family in the hospital. I could tell that my presence was a double-edged sword: showing her the reality of what she might face if she got amputations, but also offering hope for her future. Not just for her, but for her gathered family. Realizing she might need prosthetic legs like mine was shocking, but seeing me successfully navigate the world in my post-sepsis form gave them hope, and permitted them to envision a future for and with her.

If there was any question as to whether or not sharing my story was making an impact, that question had been answered with a resounding "yes!"

Walking Forward on Solid Footing

As time rolls on and I grow in confidence, competence, and knowledge, more and more opportunities arise to share what I've learned and help others navigate, or hopefully avoid altogether the harrowing territory I've tread. The legs and fingers I lost intrigue people and make them want to hear my story. My voice, despite the damage done by sepsis, grows ever stronger as I use it to speak up for those who never got the chance to share their stories.

My tragic experience has led to miracles and positive outcomes beyond my wildest imagination. I am continually humbled by the powerful mysteries of the world we live in. At the end of the day, I have nothing but gratitude for all that wasn't lost, and for all that has been found.

EPILOGUE - ONWARD

Glinda: You've always had the power..., my dear.

Tin Man: Then why didn't you tell her?

Glinda: Because she wouldn't have believed me. She had to learn it for herself.

– *The Wizard of Oz,* adapted from the book by L. Frank Baum

"Do you want to hold him?"

I froze.

I'd imagined this moment so many times. I'm standing in Queen's Medical Center – this time on the Big Island, where we're building our retirement home, and this time for the best of reasons: *to hold my first grandbaby!* I had always pictured myself graciously accepting that most precious of gifts, gently rocking back and forth and peering down at the most beautiful little face in the world, completely content.

But now that it was actually happening, I was flooded with anxiety. It was as though I'd been transported to my past traumatic days in the hospital.

My grandson's delivery was relatively smooth, but there were complications, and the medical team was keeping a close eye on my daughter. My PTSD kept whispering to me, *"They aren't out of the woods yet. What if your daughter or grandson gets an infection? It could lead to sepsis..."*

I had to keep reminding myself that just because I had been through a traumatic experience in the hospital didn't mean anything bad would happen to them. They were receiving excellent medical care, and I had been reassured that they were both being closely monitored for any signs of infection.

Still, my old nemesis, negative self-talk, continued: *What if my prosthetic legs trip over something I can't feel?* I hadn't felt this vulnerable on my legs in years. I took a deep, grounding breath and sat down.

I am safe. Dani and her baby are safe. Enjoy this moment!

From that stable position I reached out my arms, my capable hands with strong thumbs and shortened fingers outstretched, ready to receive that beautiful bundle of joy.

"Grandma Katy," my son-in-law Hunter spoke in a hushed tone as he carefully transferred the newborn from his arms to mine. "This is your grandson, Asher."

I felt his tiny, warm body wriggle against me as he settled into my arms. It was as if I had traveled back in time to the moment I held my first baby, his mother. My eyes brimmed with tears as I wiped them away to more clearly see his miraculous face.

Did Hunter and Dani know what a precious gift they were offering me in that moment? Not just by giving me a grandchild, but also by giving me a positive association with hospitals to replace the negative one that had reigned supreme for seven years. The same gift they'd offered me by getting married at our home in Hanalei, transforming it in my mind from the place I first got sepsis to the place where Dani and Hunter got married.

And our lives marched on.

I looked over at Scott, beaming with gratitude and pride. *Look what we made possible,* I thought. *We did this. Together.*

Some moments make all the struggles and challenges along the journey worthwhile, like reaching a spectacular viewpoint on a long hike. This was one of those, and the view was truly breathtaking.

I knew that moment wasn't about me. It was about Asher, his brand-new parents, and the beautiful family unit they made together. Still, I knew my presence at that monumental event meant something to everyone present. That magical moment would have been tinged with grief had I not beaten the odds and made it out of that other Hawaiian hospital room so I could be here in this one.

The Gift of Grit

One of my favorite sayings is that life is not a destination, it's a journey. I feel the same way about healing. I don't know if there will ever be a day when I feel "healed," "all better," or "over it." I'm sure my family agrees. But from this vantage point, I can look back at the journey and see how far we've all come. And it's clear to me that, because of this crazy adventure, we are all stronger, closer to one another, and more resilient than we ever thought we could be.

One thing I've learned about trauma and recovery is that it's life's way of making us grow more than we would have if everything had gone smoothly. In our daily lives, we grow in small, manageable increments. We are gently guided, step by step, to a higher level of consciousness, greater self-control, and strengthened compassion for others. But the real growth comes from overcoming the biggest challenges.

Before sepsis, my life had been relatively easy. I considered myself blessed and lucky. I had a loving family who nurtured me and encouraged me to be proud of my unique strengths and passions. I was well educated. I had only suffered minor heartache in my relationships. I married my high school sweetheart, and our life together had gone relatively smoothly.

I took great pride in helping my children become resilient by encouraging them to push themselves in athletics and academics, to enroll in summer programs abroad, and to try challenging new activities like snowboarding, surfing, and horseback riding. They were both adventurous in ways I had never been.

They could stand up for themselves with teachers and their peers when needed. They worked hard to get into their chosen universities and excelled there, both academically and as leaders. They always challenged themselves to reach beyond their comfort zones when risk was involved. If they failed, they learned from their mistakes and didn't let it get them down.

In short, they had a level of grit I didn't think I had ever developed. I feared I lacked the very resilience I had worked so hard to instill in my children.

Sep 29 - Scott & Jordan texts

Jordan: Definitely a mental adjustment but nothing we're feeling is anywhere close to what mom's feeling so we all gotta stay strong and support each other to support her. We're Graingers, we got this .

Scott: Hell yes. In the military, in heavy combat, they say, "we must go forward and we must go through it simply because we have no other choice." I like that.

Jordan: Good motto for right now.

Scott: I guess our choice is HOW we choose to go forward and through. That is up to each of us. I'm here for you and I'm stronger knowing you're here for me.

One of my best friends said it well at her holiday party, the first I had attended in a wheelchair without Scott's assistance. When her mom asked her how I was doing with my amputations and recovery, she replied, "She's doing really well."

To which her mom responded, "Well, of course she is! She's Katy!"

Keep in mind, I knew her mom on a friendly, surface level, so she mostly saw the positive, confident person I presented to the world.

My friend leaned over to me and said, "I just agreed with my mom because it was easiest, but between you and me, aren't you honestly surprised by how well you've managed this whole thing!?"

"Yes!" I exclaimed, thrilled that someone who knew me so well recognized that it had been a real challenge, one which I was managing better than I ever imagined I could. I had managed to thrive through impossible odds.

We all have so much more inner strength than we know. It's through painful challenges and obstacles that we discover them within ourselves. But we need the right mindset to find and use them.

Choosing Life

Scott - text to our daughters:

> A crisis is a time to come together and be strong. We are all affected by this event. Our challenge is having it bring us closer, not tear us apart. We will be challenged in the coming days and weeks. Let's all work on empathy, selflessness, patience, and courage. Our challenge is to be strong during the crisis. It will make us stronger after it's over. I love you both so much and I'm so proud of you.

When I woke up in the ICU to face a bleak new reality, I didn't have to look far for the inspiration to fight for my life. I could see it before me in my husband and daughters, who were committed to being by my side and getting through this with me. I saw it in the doctors, nurses, and medical staff who were so excited I had survived. I found it in my extended family and friends, who left hundreds of messages of encouragement on my Facebook page, sent texts and flowers, and spoke to me on the phone. I found it in the fact that I had already fought a monster that tried to kill me, and I had won.

I had no choice but to accept that the fight to save my hands and feet would be painful and come with no guarantees. The choice I had was how I would handle it all. Would I let it depress me and make me into a victim, or would I let it fuel me to fight harder to reclaim my happy life?

I made a conscious commitment to move forward and fight for my life and limbs. I faced the monster head-on in a way I never thought I could. Even though I hadn't built up grit and resilience, I found them when I needed them, and I was brave enough to use them to face adversity in a way I had never done before.

The only way out was through.

I couldn't save my fingers or my feet, but I could save my life. I could adjust my dreams and plans to find new opportunities for joy, which even sepsis and limb loss could not destroy.

Back in Greece, when I prayed for a purpose and passion for my later years, I never could have scripted this story. Still, I wouldn't change it because of all it has given to me, and all I have been able to share with the world. We can't dictate our lives, but we can move forward with faith and find the lives we are meant to live within the messy chaos of everything beyond our control.

One tiny step at a time.

ACKNOWLEDGMENTS

My deepest gratitude:

To my family, who never left my side and carried me through the most uncertain days of my life. You were with me every step of the way, advocating, praying, and loving me when I couldn't do those things for myself. You supported me through my recovery and made space for a new life for all of us. I was never alone in this; it happened to all of us and changed all of our lives deeply. Thank you for adapting with me and having the courage and insight to realize that we needed to heal together.

To my extraordinary medical teams across three hospitals, thank you for your skill, your urgency, and your compassion. You did more than save my life – you gave me the chance to live it fully again, and inspired me to help others as you do every day.

To my friends, who showed up in countless ways both big and small, I am forever grateful. Your support, encouragement, and presence reminded me that my family and I were never alone on this journey. You have grown with me through this experience and strengthened our bonds. I never imagined I would love and be loved by so many people this much in one lifetime.

To Sepsis Alliance and my many friends and colleagues there, for helping my family navigate sepsis and life after it, and for inviting me to serve on the Board of Directors. It's an honor to be part of the mission that once helped save my life. You have given me that new purpose I longed for before my sepsis journey began.

To the organizations, scientists, professors, government officials, and those working to improve sepsis awareness, recognition, treatment, and care. Thank you for the important work you're doing to make the world safer from sepsis.

To the Amputee Coalition, thank you for equipping my fellow amputees and me with the tools, resources, and hope to rebuild our lives. The sense of belonging and connection I found through your community, especially at the annual national conferences, has been transformative.

To the sepsis survivor community, the limb loss and limb difference community, and the many people who follow and support me on social media, thank you from the bottom of my heart. Your stories, encouragement, and shared experiences continue to inspire me and remind me what it means to rebuild a life after the unimaginable.

To the women who helped elevate my voice. To Beth and Adrienne, for your encouragement and support in helping me define who I could be as a sepsis survivor and amputee with a mission – a writer, a storyteller, and a voice for my new communities. I'm grateful to have two brilliant mentors guiding me every step of the way, helping me find the key stories, editing my writing, and improving it, but only when asked. To Jes, for seeing the potential of my story to help us raise even more awareness together than we could separately. Thank you for using your influence and experience to elevate our shared voice. To Karin, for encouraging me through the difficult final phase of the writing process, and for reviewing the medical portion of my story to ensure it was accurate. Your collective belief in my story and encouragement to write this book gave me the confidence to share it with the world.

This memoir may be mine, but it was carried, shaped, and sustained by all of you.

Katy

About the author

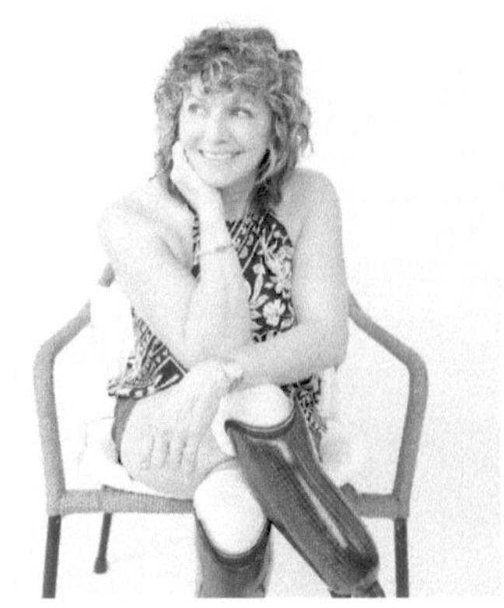

Photo by: nanikw.com

Katy Grainger was an empty nester, living in Hawaii with her husband, when her world was turned upside down by a small infection that led to septic shock and multiple amputations. Now a professional speaker, patient advocate, and sepsis educator, Katy has turned her personal trauma into a global mission. She has dedicated her life to spreading sepsis awareness, improving early detection and treatment of sepsis, empowering the limb-loss and limb-difference communities, and inspiring others that it's never too late for personal reinvention. She is a passionate member of the Board of Directors for Sepsis Alliance and Lead Advocate and volunteer for the Amputee Coalition, using her voice and experience to advance their missions.

Katy's advocacy has impacted millions. Her educational and inspirational keynote presentations have resonated with international audiences, and her viral videos have garnered millions of views, helping people worldwide recognize sepsis symptoms to save lives and better understand day-to-day life as a multiple amputee. She has been featured on major platforms, including *Women's Health*, *Amplitude Magazine*, The CDC Website, and *This Podcast Will Kill You*. She has taken her message directly to Capitol Hill to advocate for legislation supporting sepsis and amputee issues.

Married to her high school sweetheart, Katy is a proud mother of two grown daughters and recently became a grandmother to one perfect grandson. She splits her time between the Seattle area and Hawaii, prioritizing family while using her platform to prove that while sepsis may have changed her body, it could not suppress her fire.

Resources

If you found my memoir helpful or engaging, please consider:

- Leaving a review on Amazon, Goodreads, or your go-to book review space
- Purchasing *Finding Solid Footing* as a gift
- Recommending it to friends, colleagues, and loved ones

Hire me for a speaking event:

katygrainger.com/speaking

Purchase *Finding Solid Footing*:

katygrainger.com/book

Follow me on my socials: @katysepsisamputee

- Facebook Page - www.facebook.com/KatySepsisAmputee
- LinkedIn - www.linkedin.com/in/katy-grainger-752a06199/
- Instagram - www.instagram.com/katysepsisamputee
- TikTok - www.tiktok.com/@katysepsisamputee

Cover Photo Photographer - Nani Welch Keli`iho`omalu, Oahu, HI

Makeup - Tia Yagi, Hawaii Island, HI

Katy's Prosthetic Legs - Greg Davidson, Davidson Prosthetics, Puyallup, WA

Writing Resources

Beth Bornstein Dunnington's Online and Big Island Writers' Workshops - **www.bethbornsteindunnington.com**

Adrienne MacIain, Ph.D., Memoir Midwife -

https://linktr.ee/adriennemaciain

Sepsis and Amputee Resources

Sepsis Alliance - **www.sepsis.org**

Amputee Coalition - **www.amputee-coalition.org**

Enhancing Skills for Life - **www.enhancingskillsforlife.org**